High Praise for Maryann Schacht's

A CAREGIVER'S CHALLENGE: LIVING, LOVING, LETTING GO

"A Must Read! *A Caregiver's Challenge* is the friend and guide every caregiver needs. Doctors should prescribe it. Everyone trying to help someone they love through a serious illness should read it. Maryann Schacht has written an essential guide that makes a difficult time easier to survive…I wish that she had written this book 15 years ago, when my husband was dying of cancer. Her book makes a tough time immeasurably easier."
—*The Russian River Times*

"Maryann Schacht has written an outstanding book. Many authors describe the ins and outs of caregiving. Schacht does all that, and guides readers through the toughest of issues, like money, too. But she also shows us how to stay connected to life—and love—through the intense, sad, and ultimately human journey of letting go. And this is life's greatest blessing."
—Barbara Coombs Lee, President, Compassion in Dying

"Here is a sensitive, intelligent book on a role that is indeed challenging. Maryann Schacht's personal story, tracing the difficulties and triumphs in living, loving, and letting go, is woven throughout as a road map and guide. She offers a straight talking, pragmatic view of sensitive issues that come from the authority of one who has walked the path. I alternately learned from her, applauded her, and cried with her, as she moved between teacher, caregiver, and fellow traveler offering support and guidance along a bumpy road."
—Cheryl Canfield, author of *Profound Healing*

"Using both professional skills and personal experiences, Maryann Schacht creates a guidebook for caregivers."
—*The Pacific Sun*

"*A Caregiver's Challenge* is an unflinching portrait of an 'expert' facing up to her own inadequacies, defenses, illusions—all the baggage we find when reality meets theory and the process becomes personal...If you or someone you know is faced with the challenge of caring for a loved one, I would highly recommend this book as an excellent source of preparation, reference, and inspiration."
—*Sonoma Seniors Today*

"A deceptively simple book which, at first glance, is a guide for adults whose partner is dying. *Caregiver's* addresses the challenge of becoming caregiver to the one you love while (s)he is leaving you behind...A voice that is frank, funny, lyrical, pragmatic, and stubborn...She intersperses advice and wisdom culled from her deep clinical training and experience as well as from law, medicine, theology, and philosophy...Ultimately, it is this combination of self-disclosure and clinical know-how which makes *Caregiver's* so very useful for clinicians and caregivers.
—*NASW California News*

"It's a very, very pertinent book. It should be something that every rabbi, priest or minister should recommend to everybody who's suddenly in this position. It highlights all the issues that have to be dealt with—financial, emotional, medical—everything is in there. This book is very much needed."
—Rabbi Michael Robinson

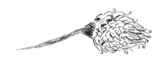

A Caregiver's Challenge:

Living, Loving, Letting Go

A Caregiver's Challenge:
Living, Loving, Letting Go

Maryann Schacht, MSW

Feterson Press
Santa Rosa, California

A Caregiver's Challenge
by Maryann Schacht

Published by:
Feterson Press
6477 Timber Springs Drive
Santa Rosa, CA 95409
(707) 537-9419
www.caregivers-challenge.net

Cover Photo © 2004 by Morris Feldman
Cover design and book layout by Judy Baker, Completely Creative

Publisher's Cataloging-in-Publication
(Provided by Quality Books, Inc.)

Schacht, Maryann.
    A caregiver's challenge: living, loving, letting go
    / Maryann Schacht.
    p. cm.
    Includes bibliographical references.
    LCCN 2004117130
    ISBN 0-9764140-0-7

    1.   Care of the sick--Psychological aspects.
    2.   Caregivers--United States--Handbooks, manuals, etc.
    3.   Helping behavior.   I. Title.
    R726.5.S33 2005   362'.0425
                                       QBI04-800144

For Bob
who taught me the meaning of courage and commitment.

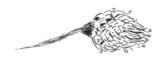

Acknowledgments

I want to thank my friends and colleagues who have encouraged me throughout the writing of this book. In particular I thank my editor Maureen Jennings, who has served as cheerleader, sounding board, and eagle eyes.

Thanks also to Judy Baker whose creative ideas sparked many of my own, Melissa Mower who spent hours copy reading, Cathy Luchetti who got me started, Arlene Mandell, Tonia Ward Singer, Jody Hoddell, Jan Cusik, Stephanie Moore, and Kathleen Winter for their reading and feedback. I also thank Maryellen Siegal, MSW, Ann Lebowitz, Ph.D., Barbara Molle, MFT, Adele Pickar, MSW, Angela Stevens, MFT, and all the members of the support groups who have met with me over the years.

A special thank you to Dr. Morris Feldman for his beautiful photography and steadfast faith in this project.

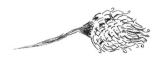

Contents

Introduction

The diagnosis has been issued. Dealing with it begins now. I wrote this book for all of you who are in that process. Many books are directed at patients, but this one addresses the problems and concerns of the well partner, the caregiver. It also explores the changing interactions that a couple facing a life-threatening illness experience. Read it together or separately. Share as much as you can.

In this day and age, as science manages to prolong life, we will all find ourselves on the seesaw. It isn't easy to balance. It requires strength and commitment and honesty. Illness challenges marriage vows and makes each of us reconsider what the word autonomy means. It is a time when all of the issues that we have managed to hide from ourselves come to the surface. Those hidden fears and emotions are shadows and they keep us from enjoying each other. We have to look at them. We have to label them. We have to wrestle with them and put them away in a box.

I had to become a caregiver. I had no choice in the matter. I never signed on to be a nurse. I never wanted to be a homebody. I have always been a restless soul and patience has never been my strong suit. In other words, I was not qualified for this job!

I was not and am not docile. I often felt shortchanged.

In spite of all my protesting and my shortcomings, I had to accept the inevitable and become the best caregiver that I could be. As a responsible wife and committed partner, I had no choice but to stand by my man. My husband and I began living and breathing in a narrow world when chronic illness became our steady companion. We lived with the knowledge that death was just around the corner, but we never knew which corner.

When I was a young girl I believed in only one side of life: the upside. I thought only of birth, growth, wonderful sights to see, and many adventures ahead. I was daring. I dove into cold lakes and scrambled up steep hills. I disregarded any scrapes and bruises I acquired along the way. More important, I avoided scary movies!

I had parents who loved and provided whatever I truly needed, a sister who shared my mischievous escapades, and a dog to lavish attention upon. My world and my life were rich, full, and protected. It was the upside!

Then when I was fourteen, illness entered our household. My ally and sister developed non-Hodgkins lymphoma. Our family went into spasm. When she died, we each fell apart in our own way. Life had unfurled its downside. We all did the best we could at that time, but each of us handled our grief solo. The life that had been sailing along on automatic pilot suddenly came to a screeching halt, leaving me gasping for breath and full of survivor guilt.

I have worked and studied for many years in order to undo the knots left behind by her death. That was the first of many life losses and, until my husband's illness, the most traumatic.

My mother never cried. She played out her misery on the piano. My father could never really see me as I was because I could never quite become his favorite child. We learned to avoid each other as much as possible.

Ours was never a family to discuss problems, and we certainly didn't talk about death, spirituality, or love in our family system. I am sure that I became interested in the way we humans act and react as a direct result of all that. I studied psychology, earned a master's degree in social work, and kept on studying. Family systems, psychodrama, hypnosis, and imagery work all fascinated me. I used it all to facilitate groups with cancer patients and with transplant patients. In the process, I made my own peace with life and death.

For many years, I handled the thought of my own death by practicing avoidance. If the subject came up, I'd simply turn my attention to other things. I never quite convinced myself that I was immortal, but I certainly felt that the world could not go on without me.

Then, as a graduate student, I was assigned to a social work internship in a hospital. Old people and young people died there! The thought of illness was no longer avoidable. I had to deal with it every day.

Sometimes, I believe the cosmos was insisting that I become more involved with end-of-life realities. I was challenged to break out of my comfortable denial.

My job was to help the family members handle grief and loss. Professionally, I began to understand the many ways in which families deal with life changes and challenges, particularly the ways in which family members show or don't show love. As they confront issues of disease and death, honesty becomes the most essential element. Without honesty there can be no peaceful resolution. Things remain unspoken. The relationship is left incomplete.

Professionally, I have been with couples as they endeavored to stay loving and helpful to each other. I have seen them as they sorted through life choices in spite of overwhelming circumstances. I have facilitated groups for people suffering from chronic pain. I recognize that they do know what is best for them. They have their own answers. They have a great deal of knowledge. Yet they often lose sight of their strengths when under pressure.

I began this book for them. I thought I had learned to accept dying was part of living, and that you couldn't have the living without the dying. That was before my husband was diagnosed. I started the workbook based on theory. Then it became personal.

It became my own experience, my pitfalls, and my triumphs. I hope you will find them helpful to you.

There is no absolute blueprint that any of us can follow when facing serious illness. Each family and each family member is unique and has to discover his or her own approach and find his or her own resolution. On-the-job training goes with the territory.

You'll find some exercises that I have used to calm anxiety and release tension throughout this book. Opportunities are offered to kindle the warmth of honest communication. There are also tools to assist you in learning about yourself. They may help you clarify your values or pinpoint the ways in which you respond to stress. Use the table of contents as a shortcut to help you traverse your own hard times. Feel free to skip around this book. If your current concern is about money, start in that chapter. If it is about dealing with and mobilizing resources, check out the chapter on gathering information. Find what you need most and use it first.

Once upon a time, doctors made house calls, and people drew strength from local family networks. There were supports to help families adjust to their changing circumstances. Now we have to establish ad hoc social support networks and manage our own medical cases. The frenetic pace of a do-it-yourself, double-career family halts abruptly when illness develops. Suddenly, it becomes necessary to redefine our thoughts and our feelings, our relationships, and our tight schedules as well. It takes a great deal of time and energy to negotiate the medical establishment, and it takes strategy and patience to arrange for child or elder care.

It can be manageable. Support systems can be mobilized, but asking for help is not an easy thing. Many of us have trouble realigning chores and roles in a systematic way. In this book, I offer you exercises and forms to help you stay on task.

I can't tell you how difficult it was for me to learn about circuit breakers, hot water systems, and tree pruning. But when my husband began to fail,

I had to take a crash course in house maintenance, anatomy, physiology, medical treatment, and patience.

We human beings are all swimming in this ocean of life together. I believe there is strength to be found in sharing our ups and downs. Recovery and well-being are about accepting and learning from whatever life dishes out. That includes asking the hard questions, making plans, and surviving in times of loss and illness.

We have to remain functional in order to be caregivers. Disappointment, loss, envy, boredom, emotional pain, confusion, and despair often seem overwhelming.

The varied thoughts and moods were (and are) all part of me. My less than perfect parts continue to surface when least expected. Each part has to be acknowledged and accepted before it can be changed. I am still working to master my disbelief, fear, anger, and confusion. I am getting a little better at recognizing which is which.

This is my story and it is your story. It is about saying hello to oneself and still giving support to the partner you love. It is about bidding goodbye to a long and comfortable relationship. This is the ultimate caregiver's challenge: to remain steady in adversity and loving throughout loss. We have to develop the ability to let go of all expectations and accept mortality, our partner's and our own.

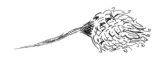

1

The Phone Call: Diagnosis

Nothing in the world lasts, save eternal change.

Honorat de Bueil, Marquis de Racan

The doctor's voice on the phone was quite clear, "I'm sorry, Maryann, but the news is not good. Your husband's biopsy shows cancer." I heard the word cancer and a shiver ran through me. I expected this, but I never believed that it would happen. It was as if I'd been hit in the stomach. I was aware of sucking in air and then I didn't feel anything at all.

Nothing moved except my breath and the words in my brain. They raced a hundred miles an hour, tripping over themselves then settling down, turning into flash cards.

No panic.

No tears. That surprised me. Usually so emotional, I was totally calm. I stared at the telephone and listened, completely numb.

I disassociated. I became quiet. I was without a trace of emotion. I was not weepy. I was not angry. I was numb. It was as if I were wrapped in some heavy plastic transparent film. Nothing hurt.

My husband was out at a meeting and not due to return for three more hours, an eternity now that time had stopped. He wouldn't be able to speak to the doctor until morning. Did I listen carefully enough? I was the one who had to tell Bob. Each word fell with a thud. What do they mean?

Old memories surfaced as my stream of consciousness went into overdrive.

Cancer haunts my family. My sister died of it. My mother died of it, breast cancer. Not the same as prostate cancer. My grandmother had colon cancer. She managed to live until she was a hundred and seven. People I love get cancer. It is a curse. My personal curse. So many friends. Friends, younger than I, no longer here. Special people. Aunt Janet, cancer of the jaw. My friends Olga and Norma died of breast cancer, much too young.

Suddenly I stopped. *Wait a minute.*

I had thyroid cancer and I am still here. I'm alive. I work with survivors of life-threatening illness all the time in my profession. I know that people recover.

I love you, Bob. There is an answer. We'll find an answer. Words rushed through my brain. A physical contraction gripped my diaphragm as if I were being punched in the stomach.

I remembered us on a camping trip when Bob was higher up the mountain than I, and he turned around and reached for my hand.

Thought upon thought strung out the theme of our togetherness, a blending polyphony observed quietly from this far-off place. My thoughts scattered and broke into shards. I observed them from my far-off place. Head chatter and images became grace notes cascading down from treble to bass clef. They tumbled off the staff.

The doctor's voice continued, "Are you all right, Maryann? Tell Bob to call me if he has questions. Here is my home number."

"Thank you, Doctor," I said, oh so graciously. "Thank you for your kindness. Thanks for your concern."

I was well-behaved, far too well-behaved.

Disassociation can be a helpful mechanism. My mother's training in manners escorted me through this stilted life-changing conversation. I was appropriate.

J.D. Londy, Ph.D. calls it a "trauma membrane." It gives a person time to decide how to cope. The body is numb but the mind races. When we humans are threatened by outside forces, the body releases catecholamines (stress hormones) into our system. The hormones prepare us to respond by choosing between two modes of behavior—fight or flight, with one sometimes more useful than the other. Wrapped in the trauma membrane, we can choose our course of action. The numbness allows time for a choice.

Just after the numbing, I expected my fight response to kick in, but it didn't happen. Was I angry? I didn't feel angry.

I was lost in intellectualization (another defense). I felt that I must write, organize, itemize, and take stock.

Make an appointment for our bone scan. It *is already "our" bone scan.*

Call the Cancer Information Hotline.

Dissipate this intensity. *Do this first.*

I dialed my sister-in-law's number in search of a way to steady myself.

Nothing could help. There was no intervention possible, at least not that night, but Myrna had always been steady. She had the precious ability to listen, and she had walked in these same shoes less than five years ago.

Her husband also had prostate cancer. She cared for him and cared about him. She was valiant. I could learn from her.

Three years my junior but definitely a role model, Myrna is more than a sister-in-law to me. She is my friend. We are both aware that in this conversation I was only occasionally rational. I felt as if I were in an art movie that had no plot. She did not comment about it, and I was enormously grateful for her tact. In my rambling I was able to displace my anxiety.

When Bob got home, I related the whole conversation to him verbatim, without breaking into tears. Bob's response was measured, rational. "We'll deal with it," he said.

"Of course," I answered.

We brushed our teeth and climbed into bed and turned away from each other, only the soles of our feet keeping our connection inviolate.

Both of us had difficulty getting to sleep.

This was the first of what would be many nights of insomnia. He solved his by taking long, hot baths and reading. He amassed information at an enormous rate. He read anything and everything: detective stories, biographies, potboilers, how to build an airplane, military strategy books, and medical papers. Some of the books just took up mind space, some informed.

I didn't do that. My mind wandered and sometimes I didn't know what I'd read, so I practiced imagery and breathing exercises. Sometimes that helped me to nod off. I found I needed to do my reading during the day. When I read late at night, my mind drifted. Meditation calmed me and, even if I didn't fall asleep, I felt more relaxed.

I am increasingly aware of my dreams. In one I'm counting numbers, 55, 72, 17. Mom died at fifty-five. Dad was seventy-two. My sister was seventeen. 55, 72, 17. Where do I fit? How much time have I got? How much time has Bob got?

It is not unusual for the patient to accept his or her diagnosis with more equanimity than the significant other. Remember the often voiced aphorism, "This hurts me more than it does you?"

The physically healthy partner begins to envision life alone. He or she cries out in pain, caught in the process of anticipatory grief. This starts in the early crisis stage and continues throughout the illness.

There I was, the doomsday kid, bemoaning my fate.

My fate? What about his fate?

Pull yourself together, I scolded myself, ashamed that I was putting concern for myself before my concern for Bob. He was the sick one! My subconscious preoccupation was with myself. How will I survive the next few months, the next few years?

I know partners of patients often obsess about the worst possible outcome. I think back to one of my former clients and how furious she was with her husband's negativity, "He buried me as soon as he heard the word metastasis, but I am alive and I have no intention of dying. He's the one who is in terrible shape. His moping depresses me."

When we are deeply hurt, we move into anger to mask the injury. Philosopher Francis Bacon describes it as "being too sensitive of hurt."

Instantly our family shape had shifted, and we had to struggle to find meaning in what had happened. My companion, my partner, was not going to be with me. Like a child trying to tame a fearful imaginary tiger in the closet, I probed and tested to see how I could handle this stunning reality.

One night I dreamed of an old friend, a doctor whom I hadn't seen in years. Suddenly, he popped into my REM cycle to tell me he was too busy. He wasn't available.

This man is the doctor who took care of my mother. He was with her when she died.

I woke up with a start, wrestling with terror, relieved that I was no longer dreaming. I commanded myself to focus, to concentrate on something, some detail, something concrete. We had to organize. We had to make lists. We would go on a macrobiotic diet. We would find an Oriental herbalist. We would exercise. *We?*

In my flurry of planning, I didn't consult Bob. I simply took control and delivered my proclamations until, not surprisingly, he objected. He was, after all, a separate human being. It was his life I was trying to manage. *He is he and I am I.* I had a hard time remembering that.

I backtracked, apologized, and explained how totally helpless I felt. I had never been good at in-between times. Bob nodded, altogether understanding. We had been together twenty-five years. He knew my style was to jump and then look. His style was to look and then jump.

He reassured me and I got annoyed with him. *What right has he to be calmer and saner than I? He has some nerve intimating that I am less adequate than he is.* Being angry and blaming him, I didn't have to face the intensity of sorrow. *How much I care for him, my lifelong love.*

Anger: what a cool defense!

During the next few days, we dealt with each other by snapping and then making up. As concerned as I was, it didn't stop me from nagging about the rumpled clothes lying on the floor of the closet. Nonsensically we argued about trivial matters—whether our dogs should be sleeping in our bedroom, who put the cat out most recently, who was supposed to clip the rose bush. In the middle of a huge harangue, we suddenly looked at each other and melted. Each of us became overly solicitous of the other.

"What do you want for dinner?" I asked gently. "I know you like Chinese."

"No, you prefer Thai. Let's go there," he deferred.

I insisted that we go Chinese because I thought that was what he really wanted.

"No" he insisted. "Thai."

I replied gently, "Chinese." I knew what he really wanted. I was mind-reading and second-guessing. It drove him crazy.

"Stop treating me like an invalid. I feel fine," he said, and he really was perfectly fine. He was the same take-charge person he was yesterday.

Nothing had changed and everything had changed. The doctor told us Bob had cancer of the prostate. He had no pain. He had no symptoms and hated to be fussed over. He had cancer. The long process of learning to accept and accommodate to living with serious illness had begun.

As Bob begins to make demands, I overdo in attempting to meet them. Sometimes I get stubborn and snap.

In my interchanges with Bob, I used denial, compensation, and projection, a regular laundry list of defenses. Worry was displaced on to whether or not Bob picked up his clothes. Preoccupation leads to denial. Comfort and normalcy are regained by engaging in inconsequential argument. Each projects his or her own ideas as to what the other wants without asking. They try to repair the damage. It turns into a regular "After you, Alphonse," "After you, Gaston," routine. We humans react in all sorts of defensive ways. Most defenses are useful. Some are not.

We pinned our deepest hopes on the doctor and endowed him with magical qualities. Idealization helped to assuage anxiety and we tended to turn over our decision-making power. *Good kids follow prescriptions, never make a fuss, and earn brownie points.*

Brownie Points? Forget it. This was Bob's life and body. He had everything at stake. He had to be his own case manager.

Regressive or not, all emotions are valid. However, needs are best met when partners identify their desires and state them in a straightforward way. All people may fall short of expectation, but whatever happens should not occur through confusion or lack of clarity.

In the throes of regression, the ill partner may try to get his needs met by feigning helplessness. In the short run, that feels easier than taking responsibility.

Helplessness is only one choice. Another is hopefulness. I talked to Bob about Brian, a teacher who developed glioblastoma, a malignant brain tumor.

Always physically fit, Brian was in his early thirties—handsome, successful, with a beautiful wife, a small son, and a sense of mission. When physicians said chemotherapy, Brian worked out an arrangement with a fellow teacher to cover his class on chemo days. He continued to coach the soccer team—Brian was not prepared to give up.

Whenever the doctors told him the prognosis was bad, he countered with, "I'll accept your diagnosis but not your prognosis."

He found a nutritionist and embraced brown rice. Along with the macrobiotic diet, he did push-ups. After six months passed, Brian was still living life to the fullest. A year passed. The doctors were amazed. Each dire prediction seemed to motivate Brian to do something more. He experimented with Chinese herbs, acupuncture, and meditation. He didn't deny the illness or its symptoms, but he refused to give up.

Brian was an exceptional patient. Two years passed and his tumor shrank, though it didn't disappear. He continued to live each day as fully as possible. He channeled inner conflict and emotion into constructive avenues of expression. Such sublimation can yield great satisfaction.

Bob listened to my tale and said, "Okay, I'll be positive but I'm not eating brown rice!"

The next day I talked to him about Sheila. Fifty-two. Breast cancer—metastasized to her bones. A lifelong athlete, she found herself walking with difficulty but still struggled to keep up at swim practice. Before cancer, she swam competitively and won often. Then, watching her power slipping away, she reset her goals. She set her heart on swimming 200 miles in the next year. She plunged into the pool every morning and set her own pace. Sometimes she would only swim half a lap. Sometimes she felt too sick to put on her swimming cap. There were days when she looked in the mirror and cried at the sight of her bald head and lack of vitality, but she set her mind on the 200 miles.

When her energy was high she swam two, three, even six laps. She swam when she wanted to swim and swam when she didn't. On December 31, she completed her 200th mile and climbed out of the pool with a huge smile on her face. Her satisfaction was enormous, her courage contagious.

She maintained that it wasn't the actualization but the process itself that brought her satisfaction.

Bob's response to Sheila's story: "Okay, I've got the message but, since I don't like swimming, I'll play duplicate bridge."

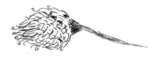

2

Who Are You after You Face Your Shadow?

You are your own friend and you are your own enemy.

Bhagavad-Gita

I heard the door slam in back. Was it Bob? The noise sounded loud. Furious? Or frustrated? Was Bob raging? Since the "illness" both of us went out of our way to tiptoe. No loud noises. No surprises, as if a startling sound could set off a terrifying round of symptoms. Maybe we overdid it, but we were careful with each other.

Bob came in looking agitated. I jumped up to comfort him, but he pushed me away impatiently. What was this? Illness? Or pent-up feelings? Did I do anything to bring this about? If so, what? Why was he so angry?

I remembered back to another time when I'd pushed his buttons. We were driving in the car—Bob was a macho man who was very proud of his driving skills. It was always important for him to be in control. We used to fight about it but then I just gave in, though I hadn't stopped being critical. So there I was, backseat driving from the copilot seat. I definitely stepped on his ego. He slammed on the brakes and declared, "That's it. I'm walking home. You think you can drive better than me? Do it. I'll walk home." He got out of the car and took off. We were miles from home.

"Hey, Bob, I'm sorry. You can't walk from here. Get back in the car."

I was in a panic. I called out the window. I apologized. He kept on walking. His behavior was over the top, but I acknowledged that he did have a right to be annoyed. That happened a long time ago. Through the years, he'd mellowed and I had mellowed. We had been through many hard times and usually we could read each other's danger signs.

That day, I didn't. There was no provocation as far I could tell. Well, it was true I did straighten up his messy desk and he didn't like that. But still, he was having a temper tantrum, raging. I thought of Jung's shadow theory. Bob's shadow was definitely out.

I don't like confrontation. It scares me. Usually, Bob operated as the ultimate pragmatist. He accepted and believed, "What is—is." But he was highly agitated and struggling to regain his composure.

Each of us has a shadow side that we do our best not to acknowledge. I like to delude myself into thinking that I know enough to recognize when mine slips out. I certainly knew when his did. It is so much easier to recognize when someone else's shadow appears.

"Maryann," he said with rising inflection, "you moved my papers. I've told you over and over not to touch my things. I can't find my appointment book. I have a doctor's appointment and I don't know when it is. Don't touch my things!"

He was furious.

What is this about? Why is he so angry? It doesn't take a genius to recognize that Bob was covering up his fear. I was afraid too.

My way of calming myself is to arrange and rearrange and put everything in order. I fuss. He charged. How would we get back on track with each other? I sensed that, if I tried to make it better, I would only make it worse. I told myself that his fury wasn't directed at me. I just needed to stay steady.

"Honey, I'm sorry. You know that I rearrange stuff when I'm nervous. I'm nervous now."

"I know," he said. "Me too." The storm was over. He reached out to me and we held each other tight.

Each of us has our own way of existing in this world. We learn various ways of coping from our families of origin, as well as from the world around us. It is not unusual for patients to accept their diagnosis with more equanimity than their mates. Remember the often-voiced aphorism, "This hurts me more than it does you"?

Bob and I differed in fundamental ways—in personality, in styles of thinking, and in behavior. As we faced stressful circumstances, we responded individually. This time I responded from the sensible adult part of me. My hurt child could just as easily have spoken up and escalated the situation.

Relationships flourish or falter because of our coping mechanisms. When styles vary, patience runs short. That certain something that drew us to our partners in the beginning becomes a trial once we fall out of lust. When the heat of first love cools, what needs to remain is caring and deep friendship.

I had always loved Bob's sense of surety, his directness, his take-charge approach to life. When we were new lovers I cherished our differences— I enjoyed his measured conclusions. He never proposed anything without weighing and measuring all the possibilities. He was the "silent man" to my "talking woman." I put my thoughts out into the universe fully aware that they were not final conclusions. He processed in his head before coming to a conclusion. He took time. I jumped right in. We were matched opposites.

When a "talking woman" slows down long enough to choose a mate, she often picks a paragon of strength and control. Is this a potential mismatch or a vital, creative, difference that stimulates the coupling?

In some cosmic approximation of dark humor, my talking everything out upset him, and his thinking everything through set off feelings of being shut out in me. I felt ignored. He felt harassed. Danger signs flashed under stress.

We want our partners to cope in the same way we do, but we also expect them to fill in our spaces. It is easy to see someone else's approach as "bad" and attempt to pressure them into doing it our way. Under stress we want them to solve problems the way that we do—if only to increase our sense of mastery. We assume that our way of coping is "right," which makes their way of coping "wrong."

I arranged things neatly and couldn't find what I was looking for. Bob used the floor for a desk and knew exactly which paper was hidden where in all his mess.

In the beginning of our marriage, we looked to each other for completion. With time, we both realized that we were both happier when we recognized our differences. We let go of our expectations. But, in our current trauma, we both forgot. We regressed into old ways of operating.

When illness intrudes on a marriage, even the strongest, most supportive environment can erode, tossing us back into the fragile expectations of our early years. In our vulnerability, we regress to recapture the innocence of youth. The patient pins a child's expectations on his or her healthy partner, who is bound to fall short. In the regressive household, the healthy partner assumes the role of the good parent offering a hug, a cookie, and the choice of TV program to the ailing partner. The patient yearns for a caretaker or guru to assume control. The caretaker cast in the role of "Father Knows Best" wants to fulfill the role, but the burden is heavy.

To psychiatrist Carl Jung, the "Human body represents a whole museum of organs, each with a long evolutionary history behind it, and we can presume that the mind is organized in a similar way."[1]

Some of our images are noble, others jealous or self-serving. Our shadows manifest the person we would be if not bound by society's rules and by conscience. They are not necessarily bad, but they are untamed.

Without shadows, we lack humanity and often energy. When we suppress them we become rigid.

For Jung our uniqueness is derived from the choices we make. We have the ability to choose how we deal with our desires. I believe that our individual temperament directs our actions. Temperaments are varied and unpredictable, developed and plucked from a bucketful of physiological, sociological, and psychological factors.

According to Jung, no one drive is more important than another. We are shadow-motivated, but we have our preferences and act accordingly. No partner can ever know all the things that were "good" in our families of origin. No one can make up for all the old hurts and difficulties once suffered.

One couple is so intent on building a life different from what they experienced in childhood that they "over bond." They allow no space for individual expression. One or the other (and sometimes both) gives up self. They become totally absorbed in each other and lose touch with the world.

They squash every difference of opinion. They sacrifice anything that might disrupt their delightful dyad. They find safety in dependency. Fear of change traps them in the status quo and robs them of spontaneity. Yet what others may see as an ironclad alliance is actually fragile circuitry, ready to shatter. Neither partner is a differentiated self. When illness intrudes, each experiences betrayal and flounders in despair.

Another couple is terrified of dependency. Each may have experienced their original families as intrusive, so they defend themselves by fighting to maintain private space. Some couples lead totally separate lives. They have little glue to bind them and under stress reside in eerie isolation, facing the change of circumstance alone.

Illness changes roles as well as rules. Familiar home life wavers and turns into a hall of mirrors. Instead of comfortable routine, there are odd reflections and strange whispers.

As the physically ill partner declines and becomes more of a burden, his concern for self grows. The healthy partner is often burdened by a frantic sense of inadequacy. *Why can't I do more? Is this the right thing? Why am I so impatient?* Worse, there is guilt about being healthy. *Why him and not me?* The nurturing spouse is called to do double duty, bending under an already staggering load. As if hallucinating, one may see the simple act of toasting waffles as alien and oppressive, or confusing and subversive. Where is stability? What is real?

The stress level created by illness is multifaceted. One partner worries about selfishness. Another worries about being disengaged. Everyone worries about drowning in a choppy sea of new requirements. While the family struggles to absorb confounding and upsetting information about the disease itself, family roles lurch back and forth like cargo in a hold, constantly sliding. The task of the family is to keep the wild pitching under control, while struggling to batten down the baggage. The family must find their balance and learn new coping skills.

Strange moods spring up. New needs make everyone uneasy. Emotions go haywire, resulting in sleeplessness and loss of energy. Worse yet, lay people have to master a new language of medicine, as well as deal with the complexity of today's health care system.

On a spiritual plane, they must come to grips with their own beliefs about life's purpose. There is no way of denying mortality. We are not immortal. The reality of death and pain hits us with a thud.

How to cope? What to do? When is the next difficulty coming?
Where to consult? Why is this happening?

Our patterns harden and set early in life. They are part of who we are. To isolate and study why we are doing *what* we are doing takes keen awareness and courage!

Stress provides us an opportunity to develop and change, but it takes determination. We must overcome childhood models. For example, if our parents reacted with panic, we may find ourselves overanxious. If the parents believed in putting the child to bed to stoically face the crisis alone, chances are that the grown-up will want solitude. Following the clue to your earliest malady can be fertile soil. Good digging.

One therapist I know asks her clients to think back to their first memory of illness. What was it like? How did your parents react? What was the solution? Prayer? Antibiotics? Isolation? Chicken soup?

Nothing brings about dysfunction like impending loss. Sharing our memories with a partner can explain present reactions and help in anticipating current responses.

We all have a continuing evolving life story. Imagine it is like a meandering ride down a jungle river. Sometimes playful monkeys swing high in the trees. Sometimes we encounter crocodiles sliding ominously into the water. A panther screams. We shudder. A bird trills and we are filled with joy. One by one the moments pass—a remarkable journey as long as we realize we are separate from the events.

We have the power to float or paddle. We can drift with the current or try paddling upstream. We can circumnavigate, head for the shore, or cross over. The journey is ours.

Native American wisdom simply says, "What is…is." The river simply is. We often want to convert "what is" into what we wish it would be.

In *I'm OK—You're OK*, author Thomas Harris says that seeing more than one point of view is the response of the mature adult who is at peace with himself or herself and others.[2]

There is no better place to appreciate "what is" than in a lifetime partnership. Here you will find the crocodiles, panthers, monkeys, and more. Do we struggle to change what we see? Make the apparitions vanish? Or do we simply relax and enjoy?

We marry because of our differences and then try desperately to make our partners over. We want them to be like us, think like us, and fill in the places of our insecurities. It is surely an oxymoron. If they acted and thought as we do, they would no longer complement us. The richness of cross-pollination would cease. If that happened, one of the two would become superfluous!

Through the centuries, thinkers have tried to unravel the mystery of our humanity. Who makes us who we are? Scientists have analyzed muscles and bones and brain matter. Social scientists have explored attraction and repulsion and social imperatives. We are still baffled by one another.

Closeness and distance change in every marriage like the tide, with successful relationships adjusting to the constant ebb and flow. Yet each time established rhythms shift and resettle, it feels terrible. *What does my partner want? Why can't he or she just tell me?* Even in the best of circumstances, relationships are bewildering. In the hard times, it takes humor to get you through.

Illness means chaos. It affects our friends and neighbors too. Some of these people will retreat, leaving us exposed and abandoned. Others take charge and direct us with lordly advice. All the retreat and/or bluster really mean is that they feel so vulnerable that they try to master an uncontrollable situation. Manager types do not like turmoil.

Carl Simonton, M.D., and Bernie Siegel, M.D., are convinced that positive engagement helps release emotional energy and helps in the healing process. Both cite the spontaneous remissions of "exceptional patients." Biologist Candace Pert, Ph.D., says, "Informational substances which have a powerful effect on mood and emotion provide a molecular way to understand the suspected connection between state of mind and state of health. Neuropeptides and lymphokines influence us on a biochemical level while imagery and emotions influence our reactions on the psychological level."[3]

What we do and how we react is directly linked to what we think and feel. The field of psychoneuroiummunology is exploding with empirical evidence. Leading scientists and theorists such as Jeanne Achtenberg, R.N., Lawrence LeShan, Ph.D., Ernest Rossi, Ph.D., Deepak Chopra, M.D., and

Larry Dossey, M.D., all point out the mind-gene connection, and the list of believers keeps growing. Meditation reinforces memories of health and well-being. We have the ability to tap into joy and remind ourselves of times when we coped effectively with adversity.

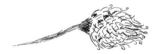

3

On Gathering Information

Tell me and I'll forget.
Show me and I may remember.
Involve me and I'll understand.

Chinese Proverb

This chapter is designed to help you take charge of the illness and get you both moving again. This is not designed as a comprehensive guide, but it will give you an indication of what resources are out there and how you can begin to access the information available.

Most of us don't know too much about illness. We avoid it as much as we can. When we are diagnosed with a disease, the label can sound like a death knell even when it is not one. Some of us become frozen. We stop thinking and acting in a coherent way. Charting direction helps put us back in control.

Because two heads are better than one, it is important for a couple to be very clear about their individual rights. When someone is feeling weak, he or she may feel intimidated by the medical system. He or she may feel too demanding or not demanding enough. Caregiver and patient need to understand and own the following.

A Patient's Bill of Rights

You have the right to:
    be comfortable with your physician.
    a second opinion (or a third).
    interview a physician.
    refuse a particular therapy.
    refuse medication.
    think things over and not rush into action.
    your anxiety.
    see your records.
    copies of letters and x-rays.
    know what side effects may come from surgery, medication, radiation, or chemotherapy.
    have a family member or other support person with you when a plan of action is being explored or explained.
    make your own decision and not to succumb to pressure.
    resist emotional blackmail.
    explore alternative therapy (herbs, acupuncture, etc.).
    remain silent.
    chatter.
    seek a support group.
    refuse a support group.
    dignity.
    grieve.
    manage your own case!

First and foremost, ask your physician for written information. Get as complete a description as possible of the diagnosis. Find out the exact name of the illness. Remember that you are the customer. There is actually evidence in the scientific community that indicates assertive patients experience less discomfort and live longer than docile patients do. So help your partner practice being assertive.

Your physician or the nurse practitioner or the social worker in the office can spend some time explaining the ramifications of your problem. Ask them. That is the key word: ask. You need to understand exactly what is going on. One of the professional staff should be able to tell you just which local hospitals have open libraries and which ones are user-friendly for patients and caregivers.

There is a flagship model library at 15891 Los Gatos-Almaden Road in Los Gatos, California, called Planetree Health Library (www.planetreesanjose.org), that has a particularly friendly approach for lay people. If you give them your diagnosis, they will bring you a file with articles that relate to it. They will do a computer search of the literature for you or help you do one. You can call them at (408) 358-5667.

If Planetree is inaccessible to you, you can start your search for information at your own local library or at a local health resource library. More are opening up every month. They are usually associated with local hospitals. County hospitals are mandated to serve the public. These libraries offer a mixture of medical books and books written for the layperson. They usually have a file of articles clipped from journals and newspapers available as well. Reference librarians are trained to track what you need and will welcome your inquiries. Many local libraries have computer links to medical libraries at universities throughout the United States.

If you are computer literate you can use the online services yourself. There is a database called InfoTrac Health Reference Center (27500 Drake Road, Farmington Hills, MI 48331) or you might try Information Access at 800-227-8431. Access to these databases can be obtained through public and college libraries, which have paid membership fees. Ask the reference librarian for help researching these databases. Don't be reticent about asking questions or asking for help.

Libraries have information in books, periodicals, and other media. So much information may feel intimidating. Don't let it be. Take a deep breath and access your determination. Once you start, you will find that it isn't so difficult after all. Most librarians love to assist. That's what they were trained to do. It is their job!

When you start talking to your local reference librarian (or your own computer), be as specific as you can. If you tell the reference librarian exactly what you are looking for, he or she will go out of his or her way to be helpful. Making your queries as detailed as possible will also help you in your computer research. If you don't have a computer at home, use one in your local library.

Do you want information on the latest medical trials or general background on the disease? Do you want statistics? Do you want to know whether there is a support group in your area?

You will find that you may have to tease your brain and think through the disease in broad terms before you zero in on a particular symptom. Try using synonyms. You may have to experiment with a number of ways of defining your subject. This vast world of information is open to you.

Those of you who are new to computers may feel overwhelmed at first. Then you may find that puzzling through is not only helpful but can also be a welcome distraction. When you become frustrated, slow down, rethink, and reframe. See your research as a quest. Knowledge is the Holy Grail and it is out there, in the keyword index. If you are going to do your own search, you must have some familiarity with the technology. If you are already an experienced surfer, you know that. If you aren't, information professionals are available to help you.

There is an Encyclopedia of Associations so you can identify groups of other people who have your same problem. Whatever you are experiencing, you are not alone. Just knowing that helps. Making direct contact with the folks who are experiencing what you are experiencing can strengthen your coping capacities.

Magazine and journal articles can be accessed via computer and you can download what you need from them. (If you are using a library, you can get a printout for a small fee.) Most university libraries are open to the public. A phone call will let you know their hours.

Medline Plus (www.medlineplus.gov) is a database that can be accessed by computer. The site covers over 650 health topics and is provided as a service of the U.S. National Library of Medicine and the National Institutes of Health. You'll find journal articles, research developments, and advice on drugs. It gives the information in English and Spanish. You ought to be able to find what you are looking for by accessing that.

If you are interested in alternative healing, there is a book out called *Alternative Healing: The Complete A-Z Guide to More than 150 Alternative Therapies* by Mark Kastner, L.Ac., Dipl.Ac., and Hugh Burroughs (ISBN 0963599712). It is published by Halcyon Publishing Co., P.O. Box 4157, La Mesa, CA 91944-4157. *The New York Times Guide to Alternative Health,* by Jane E. Brody and Denise Grady (ISBN 0805067434), published by Times Books (2001), also provides good information.

Two other resources are *Alternative Medicine Yellow Pages* by Melinda Bonk (ISBN 0963633422), published by Future Medicine Publishing (1994) and *Alternative Medicine: The Definitive Guide 2nd Edition* by Burton Goldberg et al (ISBN 1587611414), published by Ten Speed Press (2002). There are many more current online resources, including the National Center for Complementary and Alternative Medicine (www.nccam.nih.gov) and the Alternative Medicine Foundation (www.amfoundation.org).

Ask questions. Keep on asking questions. When you take control of your case, you take control of your choices. The more informed you are, the more options you have. Get to know your doctor. Ask what he or she would do if you were incurable. Ask if your requests for no artificial life support would be honored. How would he or she feel about keeping you on full life support? Ask the doctor how he or she feels about you going to a specialist and if he or she would be able to recommend one. When two of you are present at the interview, one of you will remember exactly what has been said. Don't be afraid to take notes. Write down a list of questions before you visit the doctor.

Becoming knowledgeable about the illness enables you to become partners in your care. It does not mean that you become your own doctor. But you are the persons most concerned. If you read and gain some understanding, you may be able to bring something to your physician's attention that might otherwise have been overlooked.

Suggestions

Start your own file. Start a notebook and jot down comments and thoughts. Write down requests and bequests. When it is in writing, you can feel that your wishes (or your spouse's wishes) are being followed. A notebook will take the guessing out of your decision-making. We all forget important concerns under pressure. When they are written down, we are less likely to walk out of the doctor's office with questions unanswered. When you formulate your questions, you may consider sending them along to the doctor before your appointment. That will give him or her a chance to think about them. Physicians are people too. They can't know everything. Having the opportunity to review your questions gives the doctor time to research, consider, and respond thoughtfully. That's a win-win situation.

Make sure to keep letting your doctor in on your thinking. You want your physician to be a partner. You want him or her to always work on your behalf. You want him or her to be able to honor your wishes and you want to know when he or she won't or can't do that.

Keep all your records and doctor's correspondence in a file. Make sure that copies of tests and physician opinions are sent to you. It is surprising how long it takes for information to be transcribed. All too often, we show up for a consultation only to find that important information is "still in the mail." You want to have the information ready and available. Some doctors may find your assertiveness difficult to handle, but that is their problem. If your doctor is put out, that is good information for you. If your physician is not open to your queries, find yourself another physician.

Because illness renders us so vulnerable, it is most important to keep reminding ourselves that personal autonomy is written into our American heritage. Every schoolchild is taught that he or she has the right to life, liberty, and the pursuit of happiness. It is up to us to get in touch with that pursuit. Each of us has the right to walk our own path. This right applies to health care too.

"No right is held more sacred, or is more carefully guarded than the right of every individual to the possession and control of his own person, free from all restraint or interference of others, unless by clear and unquestionable authority of law." (Union Pacific v. Botsford, 1891).

Judge Benjamin Cardozo declared, "Every human being of adult years and sound mind has a right to determine what shall be done with his own body; and a surgeon who performs an operation without his patient's consent commits an assault." (Schloendorff v. New York Hospital, 1914).

In the 1983 Nancy Cruzan case, the Supreme Court declared that each of us has the right to make health care decisions from our "liberty interest" even when we become incapacitated, if there is clear and convincing evidence that the decision is the patient's wish. Make sure you put your wishes in writing! See Chapter 12 for a sample directive.

We have legal precedence, which says that you have the right to take charge of your health. It is your life to live as fully as possible.

More Resources to Get You Started

AIDS Research Alliance of America
621-A No. San Vicente Blvd.
West Hollywood, CA 90069
(310) 358-2423
www.aidsresearch.org

AIDS Survival Project
139 Ralph McGill Blvd., Ste. 201
Atlanta, GA 30308
(877) AIDS-444
www.aidssurvivalproject.org

Alzheimer's Association
225 N. Michigan Ave., Ste. 1700
Chicago, IL 60601-7633
(800) 272-3900
(312) 335-8700
www.alz.org

Alzheimer's Disease Education *&*
Referral (ADEAR) Center
National Institute on Aging
P.O. Box 8250
Silver Spring, MD 20907-8250
(800) 438-4380
www.alzheimers.org

American Brain Tumor Association
2720 River Road
Des Plaines, IL 60018
(800) 886-2282
(847) 827-9910
www.abta.org

AMC Cancer Research Center
1600 Pierce St.
Denver, CO 80214
(800) 321-1557
www.amc.org

American Cancer Society
(800) 227-2345
www.cancer.org

American Diabetes Association
Attention: National Call Center
1701 N. Beauregard St.
Alexandria, VA 22311
(800) 342-2383
www.diabetes.org

American Heart Association
National Center
7272 Greenville Ave.
Dallas, TX 75231
(214) 373-6300
www.americanheart.org

American Kidney Fund
6110 Executive Blvd., Ste. 1010
Rockville, MD 20852
(800) 638-8299
www.kidneyfund.org

American Liver Foundation
75 Maiden Lane, Ste. 603
NY, NY 10038
(800) GO-LIVER
liverfoundation.org

American Lung Association
61 Broadway, 6th Floor
NY, NY 10006
(212) 315-8700
www.lungusa.org

American Osteopathic Association
142 E. Ontario St.
Chicago, IL 60611
(800) 621-1773 or (312) 202-8000
www.osteopathic.org

American Parkinson's
Disease Association, Inc.
1250 Hylan Blvd., Ste. 4B
Staten Island, NY 10305
(800) 223-2732
www.apdaparkinson.org

American Speech-Language-
Hearing Association
10801 Rockville Pike
Rockville, MD 20852
(800) 638-8255
www.asha.org

American Stroke Association
(A division of the American Heart
Association)
www.strokeassociation.org

American Stroke Foundation
11902 Lowell
Overland Park, KS 66213
(913) 649-1776
www.americanstroke.org

Association for the Care
of Children's Health Network
19 Mantua Road
Mt. Royal, NJ 08061
(609) 224-1742

Brain Injury Association of America
8201 Greensboro Dr., Ste. 611
McLean, VA 22102
(703) 761-0750
(800) 444-6443 Family Helpline
www.biausa.org

Cancer Information and
Counseling Line
(800) 525-3777
or email ciclhelp@amc.org

Cancer Information Service
National Cancer Institute
(800) 422-6237
(1-800-4-CANCER)
cis.nci.nih.gov

Cancervive, Inc.
11636 Chayote St.
Los Angeles, CA 90049
(800) 4-TO-CURE
(310) 203-9232
www.cancervive.org

CDC National HIV
and AIDS Hotline
(800) 342-2437
They do not give out their address.
Please call and they will send you
information.

Children Affected by AIDS
Foundation
6033 W. Century Blvd. Ste. 280
Los Angeles, CA 90045
(310) 258-0850 and
5315 N. Clark Street, Ste. 310
Chicago IL 60640
 (773)588-0075
www.caaf4kids.org

Elton John AIDS Foundation
P.O. Box 17139
Beverly Hills CA 90209-3139
Voice Mail (310) 535-1775
www.ejaf.org

I Can Cope
(A program of the American
Cancer Society)
(800) 227-2345

International Association for the
Study of Pain
909 NE 43rd St., Ste. 306
Seattle, WA 98105
(206) 547-6409
www.iasp-pain.org

International Association of
Laryngectomees
P.O. Box 691060
Stockton, CA 95269-1060
(866) 425-3678
www.larynxlink.com

Leukemia & Lymphoma Society
1311 Mamaroneck Ave.
White Plains, NY 10605
(914) 949-5213
www.leukemia-lymphoma.org

Lupus Foundation of America, Inc.
2000 L St., NW, Ste. 710
Washington, D.C. 20036
(202) 349-1155
www.lupus.org

Mended Hearts, Inc.
7272 Greenville Ave.
Dallas, TX 75231-4596
(888) 432-7899
www.mendedhearts.org

National Association
for Continence
P.O. Box 1019
Charleston, SC 29402-1019
(800)BLADDER
www.nafc.org

National Association of People
with AIDS
1413 K St. NW, Ste. 700
Washington, D.C. 20005
(202) 898-0414
www.napwa.org

The National Breast Cancer
Coalition
1101 17th Street NW, Ste. 1300
Washington, D.C. 20036
(800) 622-2838
www.natlbcc.org

National Coalition for
Cancer Survivorship
1010 Wayne Ave., Ste. 770
Silver Spring, MD 20910
(877) 622-7937
www.canceradvocacy.org

National Heart, Lung and Blood
Institute Health Information Center
P.O. Box 30105
Bethesda, MD 20824-0105
(301) 592-8573
www.nhlbi.nih.gov

National Institute of Allergy and
Infectious Diseases
Building 31, Room 7A-25, 31
Center Drive MSC 2520
Bethesda, MD 20892-2520
(301) 496-5717
www.niaid.nih.gov

National Institute of Arthritis and
Musculoskeletal and Skin Diseases
Information Clearinghouse
1 AMS Circle
Bethesda, MD 20892-3675
(877) 266-4267
www.niams.nih.gov

National Institute of Diabetes and
Digestive and Kidney Diseases
Information Clearinghouse
    Diabetes:
    (800) 860-8747
    Digestive diseases:
    (800) 891-5389
    Kidneys and Urology:
    (800) 891-5390
www.niddk.nih.gov

National Multiple Sclerosis Society
733 Third Ave.
NY, NY 10017
(800) 344-4867
www.nmss.org

National Organization for
Rare Disorders
P.O. Box 1968
Danbury, CT 06813-1968
(800) 999-6673
www.rarediseases.org

National Stroke Association
9707 E. Easter Lane
Englewood, CO 80112
(800) STROKES
www.stroke.org

Operation Stroke (Affiliated with
American Heart Association)
7272 Greenville Avenue
Dallas, TX 75231
(888) 4-STROKE
www.strokeassociation.org

Stroke Clubs International
805 Twelfth St.
Galveston, TX 77550
(409) 762-1022

The Stroke Information Directory
www.stroke-info.com

Survivors c/o American Foundation
for Suicide Prevention
120 Wall St., 22nd Floor
NY, NY 10005
(888) 333-2377
www.afsp.org

United Ostomy Association, Inc.
19772 MacArthur Blvd., #200
Irvine, CA 92612-2405
(800) 826-0826
www.uoa.org

Y-ME National Breast Cancer
Organization
212 W. Van Buren, Ste. 500
Chicago, IL 60607
(312) 986-8338
(800) 221-2141 Hotline
www.y-me.org

Please remember that phone numbers and addresses do change. Please feel free to check my website www.caregivers-challenge.net for current information.

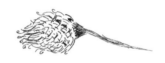

4

Managing Pain: Focus and Imagery

Pain has an element of blank. It cannot recollect.
When it began, or if there were a day when it was not.

Emily Dickinson

The hardest days were the ones when I knew Bob was suffering and his stoic attitude drove me crazy. I felt so helpless. I knew it didn't have to be. Physicians know how to make a patient comfortable but society indoctrinates us. Drug addiction is BAD. Boys mustn't be sissies. It is difficult to change a long-held pattern.

When it hurts it hurts, but how much you allow pain to take over your life has a great deal to do with being able to get the help you need. This chapter is all about pain and will offer a variety of coping strategies that have proven to be helpful and useful to others.

Response to pain is individual and has only a little to do with your character structure. Obviously, if someone is anxiety ridden, fearfulness will magnify pain sensations. Stoicism and bravado may be useful, but they often mask clues that could enable a physician to get the patient the needed relief. Sometimes intense physical pain clouds the mind and makes it hard to describe just what is going on. It is challenging to find words to describe what one feels. Pain is hard to define and describe.

A patient may wonder if he or she complains too much or too little. What each individual feels is not relative to what anyone else experiences. Comparison should never be an issue. Each of us is entitled to feel in his or her own way.

Consider identifying the pain by placing it on a scale from 0 to 10, using 0 as feeling pain free and 10 as the pain feeling intolerable. Let the doctors and nurses know how it is experienced in this moment. Make sure that a pain inventory is given to the doctor.

It is agonizing to see someone you love in pain. You feel powerless and frustrated. You want to do something, anything.

Copy the inventory on the following page and ask your patient to fill it out. Do this often.

The physician and the patient will find it useful. It also gives you something tangible to help overcome your feelings of helplessness.

Brief Pain Inventory

Today's Date _____ Date of Birth _____

First Name _____ Middle Name _____

Last Name _____

Area Code _____ Phone Number _____

1. Marital State (at present)

    a. Single   b. Married   c. Widowed   d. Divorced

2. Education (Circle the highest degree completed) Grade

0	1	2	3	4	5	6	7	8	9
10	11	12	13	14	15	16	M.A./M.S.	Professional Degree	

3. Current Occupation _____
    (Specify titles: if you are not working, tell us your previous occupation)

4. Spouse's Occupation _____

5. Which of the following best describes your current job status

    a. Employed outside the home full time

    b. Employed outside the home part time

    c. Homemaker

    d. Retired

    e. Unemployed

    f. Other

6. How long has it been since you learned your diagnosis? _____ Months

7. Have you ever had pain due to your present disease?

   a. Yes   b. No   c. Uncertain

8. When you first received your diagnosis was pain one of your symptoms?

   a. Yes   b. No   c. Uncertain

9. Have you had surgery in the last month?

   a. Yes   b. No   c. Uncertain

10. Throughout our lives, most of us have pain from time to time (such as minor headaches, sprains and toothaches). Have you had pain other than these everyday kinds of pains in the last week?

    If you answered yes to the last question, please go on to question 11 and finish this questionnaire. If no, you are finished with the questionnaire.

11. On the diagram (on the next page) shade the areas where you feel pain. Put an X on the area that hurts most.

12. Please rate your pain by circling the one number that best describes your pain at its worst in the last week.

0	1	2	3	4	5	6	7	8	9	10
No Pain										Pain as bad as you can imagine

13. Please rate your pain by circling the one number that best describes your pain at its least in the last week.

0	1	2	3	4	5	6	7	8	9	10
No Pain										Pain as bad as you can imagine

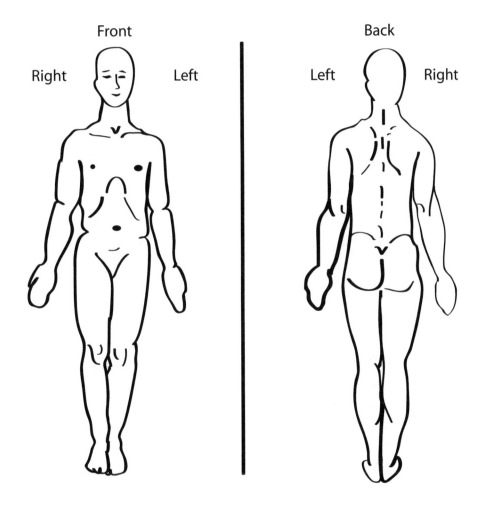

14. Please rate your pain by circling the one number that best describes your pain on average.

0	1	2	3	4	5	6	7	8	9	10
No Pain										Pain as bad as you can imagine

15. Please rate your pain by circling the number that tells how much pain you have right now.

0	1	2	3	4	5	6	7	8	9	10
No Pain										Pain as bad as you can imagine

16. What kinds of things make your pain feel better (for example, heat, medicine, rest)?

17. What kinds of things make your pain feel worse (for example, walking, standing, lifting)?

18. What treatments or medications are you taking for your pain?

_____

19. Please circle the one percentage that shows how much relief you have received in the last week.

0%	10%	20%	30%	40%	50%	60%	70%	80%	90%	100%
No Relief										Complete Relief

20. If you take pain medication, how many hours does it take before the pain returns?

    a. Pain medication doesn't help at all hours

    b. One hour

    c. Two hours

    d. Three hours

    e. Four hours

    f. Five to twelve hours

    g. More than twelve hours

    h. I do not take pain medication

21. Circle the answer for each item.

    I believe my pain is due to:

    a. The effects of treatment (for example, medication, surgery, radiation, prosthetic device).

       ☐ Yes   ☐ No

    b. My primary disease (meaning disease currently being treated and evaluated).

       ☐ Yes   ☐ No

    c. A medical condition unrelated to primary disease (for example, arthritis).

       ☐ Yes   ☐ No

22. For each of the following words, check yes or no if that adjective applies to your pain.

Aching	☐	Yes	☐	No
Throbbing	☐	Yes	☐	No
Shooting	☐	Yes	☐	No
Stabbing	☐	Yes	☐	No
Gnawing	☐	Yes	☐	No
Sharp	☐	Yes	☐	No
Tender	☐	Yes	☐	No
Burning	☐	Yes	☐	No
Exhausting	☐	Yes	☐	No
Tiring	☐	Yes	☐	No
Penetrating	☐	Yes	☐	No
Nagging	☐	Yes	☐	No
Numb	☐	Yes	☐	No
Miserable	☐	Yes	☐	No
Unbearable	☐	Yes	☐	No

23. Circle the number that describes how, during the past week, pain has interfered with your:

a. General Activity

0	1	2	3	4	5	6	7	8	9	10
Does not interefere										Completely interferes

b. Mood

0	1	2	3	4	5	6	7	8	9	10
Does not interefere										Completely interferes

c. Walking Ability

0	1	2	3	4	5	6	7	8	9	10
Does not interefere										Completely interferes

d. Normal Work (includes work outside the home and housework)

0	1	2	3	4	5	6	7	8	9	10
Does not interefere										Completely interferes

e. Relations with Other People

0	1	2	3	4	5	6	7	8	9	10
Does not interefere										Completely interferes

f. Sleep

0	1	2	3	4	5	6	7	8	9	10
Does not interefere										Completely interferes

g. Enjoyment of Life

0	1	2	3	4	5	6	7	8	9	10
Does not interefere										Completely interferes

Charles S. Cleeland, M.D., Pain Research Group, University of Wisconsin Medical School.[4]

If pain is not appropriately addressed, it causes emotional as well as physical suffering. As a patient, your willingness to explain and explore alternatives will help you find something that is particularly soothing and useful to you. In order to get the relief you want, you have to be demanding. You have to be your own advocate. Every day new approaches are being discovered. Analgesics can help. Relaxation techniques can help. Distraction can help. Just keep reminding yourself that you have a right to relief, so keep asking for it and trying different approaches.

The first step is to zero in on what you are feeling and where you are feeling it in your body. Your physician will probably ask you to develop a pain history but, if he or she doesn't, fill out the following page and bring it in yourself.

Pain History

1. How do you react to pain?

2. What do you do to handle minor pain?

3. Have you taken pain medication in the past?

4. If so, what did you take? How often? How much? How long?

5. Did you have a reaction?

6. Is your pain chronic?

7. Does anything besides medication help decrease your pain?

8. Is your pain interfering with your home life, job, school, or social life?

9. Are you experiencing depression? Anxiety? Other negative feelings?

10. Is there anything that needs to be recorded on your medical chart?

11. Do you use any over-the-counter drugs to counteract your pain? Is it effective?

12. Do you have any fears about pain, pain medication, opioids, or other drugs? Is there anything that you don't want to try? Why?[5]

Other Things to Try

Keeping a pain diary is helpful and another area in which the whole family can work together. The person experiencing the pain may not be aware of causative factors, although an observant partner can pinpoint what is contributing to dis-ease by helping with the pain diary. The more specific this record is the better.

If there is anything that alleviates the intensity of your pain, write it down. Sometimes a shift in position helps. Sometimes heat or ice helps. Write down in the pain diary your observations on the hours you have slept or not slept. A description of your affect and mood as well as what was transpiring in the room at the time will help shed light on the situation. List what relaxation techniques you tried and report their outcome. Think about anything that interrupted your focus or anything that helped you to concentrate. Sometimes details that seem insignificant are just the clues that become the most helpful.

A number of non-drug approaches can help. Neuropeptides released from the brain can quiet or excite all parts of the system. Your thoughts have the power to turn on your opiate receptors and release tiny endorphins throughout your system. Endorphins are the body's natural opiates. Through the use of imagery, you can quiet pain or exacerbate it. You can truly be your own drugstore. Just as you used focusing to help isolate a problem, you can also use relaxation/meditation to lessen pain.

It may be helpful to study a diagram indicating where the receptors are located in the brain and place your attention on those sites during your relaxation meditation.[6]

Find a comfortable and quiet spot. Try placing a pillow under the small of your back or under a throbbing arm. The cushioning may enable you to find a more comfortable position. Sometimes a heating pad or an ice pack placed under the sore area will help you to relax. Allow yourself to become as quiet as possible.

The following exercises will help you focus and distract you from your pain at the same time.

The Staircase

Begin to breathe deeply and evenly. Slowly imagine yourself walking down a flight of stairs and as you descend counting backwards from 10 to 1. Breathe. Inhale. Exhale. Breathe slowly and evenly and now notice the air as it leaves your nostrils.

Send the breath slowly into your head and into your cheekbones and into your jaw. Breathe into your neck and relax whatever tension is there. Breathe into your shoulders and relax. Breathe into your upper back and relax. Breathe into your arms all the way to your fingertips.

Breathe into your lower back and your belly. Breathe into your liver and your intestines. Breathe into the area around your genitals and now breathe into your thighs, your knees, and your calves. Breathe into your ankles and your heels and your toes. Feel how relaxed you are now. Feel how calm you are.

Try changing the clear color of your exhaled air into the color red and as you do, breathe out the pain. Watch the red vapors of pain leaving your body. Let go of the pain. Concentrate on exhaling the pain. Send the red vapors upward and transform them into orange swirls. Breathe out and let them go on their way.

If you are ready, play with changing those orange vapors into yellow vapors and let them drift away as well. Watch them go. Let them go.

As they drift away, imagine green healing clouds forming. You may want to inhale the green moisture. Green is a healing color. Stay with the greening as long as you wish. Breathe in. Exhale. Breathe in. Exhale. Breathe at your own pace.

Here at this healing level is an opportunity to address your pain. Allow it to take shape and form. Introduce yourself to your pain and acknowledge that it is alerting you, warning you of anything amiss in your system. Appreciate that it is working on your behalf. As you listen to the pain, take note of its size and shape. Acknowledge its existence. Breathe with it. Breathe into it. Breathe around it.

You might even want to thank it for trying to help you identify your difficulty. Ask if the pain would be willing to discuss the situation with you. Ask it what it is trying to tell you and listen to the answer.

Ask it what it needs in order to allow you to become more comfortable. Breathe in the soothing healing green vapor and, as you exhale, slowly change the color to blue. Deep, deep, blue. Breathe in the coolness. Let it move throughout your body. Take as much time with it as you need and then imagine the blue changing and becoming darker and deeper until it becomes purple. Dark, dark, purple.

Allow it to fill you up with quiet and sense the richness that is your true essence. Breathe with the purple. Float on the waves of purple. Take as much time as you need. When you find yourself free and calm, imagine yourself returning to the staircase, and count yourself up from your dreaming.

Climb step 1, bringing your calmness with you, and step 2, feeling relaxed, and climb to step 3.

Counting as you go, ascend steps 4 and 5 and 6. Notice the light on your eyelids bringing your sense of well-being with you as you become conscious of your breathing. Now mount steps 7 and 8 and 9, and as you do allow yourself to become more aware of the sounds around you.

Arriving at the top step 10, let your eyes open slowly. Come back slowly, taking all the time you need to reenter this everyday world.

Note: If you reenter too quickly, you may want to close your eyes again and breathe yourself back into serenity with deep even breaths.

This kind of relaxation takes a bit of practice, but it will work. Decide to work at it. Practice at least twice a day. No self-criticism allowed! Be gentle with yourself.

Visualizing is easy for some people, but others don't see pictures. They work better in the auditory mode. If you are an "ear" person, imagine the sound of the vapor as it leaves your body. Substitute sounds for color. Experiment with tones or rhythms. Alter them. Picture them rising up a scale. Try a drumbeat and change it to a wailing saxophone, a bass fiddle, or a sweet violin.

You may be a touch person. Use that as a key. If you are a tactile person, try remembering the feel of sharpness and with each breath change the feeling until it has the softness of velvet.

The object is to recognize that you have the power to alter the way you experience what is happening. Your mind can help you accomplish marvelous feats.

Glove Anesthesia

David Bresler, Ph.D., L.Ac., a founder of the Academy for Guided Imagery, developed the technique called "glove anesthesia," designed to prepare you for dealing with pain.[7] You can use it whenever the pain is intense or when it is difficult to create your own imagery. Allow your partner to read the following script to you slowly and listen and follow the instructions as he or she does. Doing the exercise together will be helpful to both of you.

Take your time. This is a two-step exercise, and by using it you will find that you are able to develop numbness in your hand and transfer the numbness to the place that hurts.

First stretch your fingers apart as far as you can. As you do you will start to notice that feelings of numbness are already beginning to develop. You have that ability. Now get yourself into a comfortable position. Hang up a "Do not disturb" sign and take the telephone off the hook.

Take a few slow abdominal breaths. Inhale. Exhale. Inhale. Exhale.

Focus your attention on your breathing and recognize how easily slow deep breathing can help produce a state of deep and gentle relaxation.

Let your body breathe itself, according to its own natural rhythm, slowly, easily, and deeply. Now close your eyes and begin the exercise with a single breath, a special message that tells your body that you are ready to enter a state of deep relaxation. Exhale. Let out all the air in your lungs. Breathe in deeply through your nose and blow out through your mouth.

You may notice a kind of tingling sensation as you do this. Whatever you feel is your body's way of acknowledging the experience of relaxation, comfort, and peace of mind that awaits you.

Now imagine that a small table is being placed in front of you. On the table is a bucket filled with sparkling clear odorless fluid. Can you see it in your mind's eye? Is the bucket metal or plastic? What color is the bucket? Imagine it as vividly and completely as you can.

Imagine that the fluid in the bucket is an extremely potent anesthetic, one so powerful it can easily penetrate any living tissue and quickly render it insensitive to all feeling. In a moment pick up your right or left hand and then dip it to wrist level into the imaginary bucket. Really do it, really lift your hand, for if you proceed through these actions as if they were real, you may be surprised to discover that the relief that you feel will be real. Now slowly raise your hand and dip it deeper in the bucket. Notice when your fingertips begin to tingle. You are absorbing the anesthetic. When you feel the tingle or notice any change in your fingertips, slowly dip your hand deeper. Feel the numbness go to your knuckles, across your palm and the back of your hand, and now all the way up to your wrist.

The skin on your hand may be beginning to feel constricted and tingly and, as the anesthetic penetrates even deeper, you may notice a numb, wooden-like feeling in the muscles of your hand and fingers. As the numbness seeps even deeper, the bones themselves may lose all feeling. Gently swirl your hand around to ensure the deepest possible penetration of the anesthetic solution. Sense any remaining feelings in your hand moving out the tips of your fingers, floating down softly to the bottom of the bucket.

Continue to swirl your hand around for as long as it takes to achieve total anesthesia, a deep feeling of tingling numbness.

In a moment, at the count of three, remove your hand from the bucket and place it on the part of your body that hurts. This will permit you to transfer the numbness from your hand to the area of your discomfort, and, in exchange, any feeling of discomfort, tension, or tightness will flow back from this area into your hand. You will then dip your hand into the bucket again to remove the uncomfortable sensations and refill your hand again with pain-relieving numbness.

One-Two-Three. Now remove your hand from the bucket and place it directly on the part that hurts. Imagine all the deep feelings of numbness from your hand streaming into every cell of that area and simultaneously picture your hand beginning to absorb all the discomfort from that area.

Notice that the same numbness that quickly developed in your hand is now permeating the painful part of your body. Can you sense the skin constricting? Are the muscles losing all feeling as the numbness penetrates deeper? Can you experience your hand becoming filled with uncomfortable sensations you once experienced only in that affected area? Slowly rub your hand around the area until you feel you have transferred as much anesthesia and absorbed as much discomfort as you can. You may be surprised to notice how much difference this has made.

Now dip your hand once again into the bucket and repeat the exercise. Swirl your hand around in the anesthetic solution to allow the transferred feeling of discomfort to drain out through your fingertips and flow down to the bottom of the bucket.

At the same time, feel your hand react once again to the anesthetic solution, deeply absorbing it through the skin to the muscles and bones.

Once again, fill your hand completely with the feeling of tingling numbness. It will probably take less time to achieve this state than it did the last time, but continue to swirl your hand around for as long as it takes, whether it is a few seconds or even a minute or more.

Soak up as much numbness as your hand can hold and, when you are ready, place your hand back on the area of discomfort.

Once again, let the tingly, relaxed feeling of numbness seep deeply into every cell in the area. If there is any remaining discomfort, drain it back into your hand. Gently rub your hand over the area, transferring these feelings as fully as you can, until you are ready to dip your hand into the bucket once again and repeat the process.

Continue to move back and forth from the bucket to the affected area at your own pace. Each time that you repeat it, you will be able to experience an even greater amount of comfort and relief in the affected area. Each time you repeat the transfer, it will become easier and easier for you. Continue now at your own pace.

And when you are ready to end this exercise, simply shake your hand briskly and return all the feelings that you had in it before the exercise began.

After completing this exercise of glove anesthesia, you may be surprised to notice that you feel not only relaxed and comfortable, but also energized with such a powerful sense of well-being that you will be able to meet any demands that may arise.

Now open your eyes and take a single breath, exhale, breathe deeply through your nose, blow out through your mouth, and be well.

Some people find that doing arithmetic or working on crossword puzzles helps to distract them from pain. Some people turn up the volume on the TV or stereo. Do whatever works. You can often break the pain cycle by placing your attention somewhere else.

Another quick way to do this is to imagine a radio knob. Turn it to the frequency of your pain. Focus on turning the volume down. As the volume goes down, so does the pain. Breathe deeply and feel well.

Note that caregivers often suffer stress pain. They sometimes develop backaches, or headaches and/or muscle strains. Caregivers benefit from imagery work just as much as patients do.

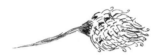

5

Where Is My Miracle?
Exploring Complementary Therapy

In spite of the cost of living, it is still popular.

Kathleen Norris

A question not to be asked is a question not to be answered.

Robert Southey: The Doctor XII

Once someone gets sick, advice pours in from every direction. Everybody you know starts telling you anecdotes about someone who was cured (or not cured) by nutrition, acupuncture, biofeedback, Chinese herbs, hypnosis, or by waving crystals. Everybody means well, but you may find yourself wishing they all would just leave you both alone. It sometimes feels as though people think that you left your judgment at the circus and your intelligence behind the barn.

One of our sons called to tell us that a clairvoyant he knew in England had told him Bob did not have cancer at all. She believed he had taken a blow to his immune system and should be taking a series of herbs and potions. Maybe she was right. Who knows? However, we both felt that a long-distance diagnosis, not test-based, was more than we could handle.

I am a great believer in imagery tapes. I have used them with clients for years, but Bob was an engineer, and he wanted and needed to read all sorts of literature before he attempted anything new. He felt this way in spite of his knowing that I had successfully used auto-hypnosis with clients for years.

Figuring that he didn't want me telling him what to do and how to do it, I chose a tape with a soothing male voice. I suggested he simply try it and then went into the office and closed the door. After a bit, I couldn't resist checking on how it was going. I found him half-listening and reading a book at the same time! I lost my cool and yelled at him, then went back into my office. I slammed the door behind me.

A few minutes later I heard the tape. I waited, ashamed of my behavior but curious. After about twenty minutes, I sneaked back into the living room. The tape was still going but I didn't see Bob. Then I heard a snoring sound and followed it. There he was in the upstairs hallway—sound asleep.

Meditation tapes were not for him!

Some of the advice people offer sounds fine. Some, though certainly well-intentioned, just doesn't fit with your particular belief system. Some of the advice is alien, but you are tempted to learn a bit more about it. Some advice seems to shout, "Try me." Don't discount your intuition. Listen to it.

All of this can be confusing, annoying, and sometimes downright discouraging. However, if you make the attempt to sort through the why's and wherefore's of the various therapies, you can come up with a plan that complements your allopathic medical program.

Acupuncture

What is acupuncture? It is a Chinese healing system 5,000 years old. While not a cure for all things, when someone with experience practices acupuncture, it may help to put the body back into a state of balance.

Acupuncture is based on the idea that specific channels are distributed like highways throughout the body. Each separate pathway is linked to its own set of organs and tissues. The vital force of energy, called chi, travels throughout the network.

Each meridian conducts its energy flow toward one of the main organs. When needles are inserted at designated acupuncture points, they change the flow of energy and pull it toward or away from the organs. The miniature shock finds its corresponding point on the surface of the body. It interrupts the chi and forces it to flow more freely.

According to Chinese thought, everything is based on yin and yang, the two polarities, plus five elements (wood, fire, earth, metal, and water).

The belief is that human beings live and interact within nature. Nothing is ever static and every object has within it two opposing energy forces, which conflict with each other and yet are totally interdependent. When you are sick, your energy (or chi) is out of balance. There is either too much yin or too much yang.

Yin is cold. Yang is hot. Contemplation is yin. Activity is yang. There is no such thing as an absolute, because everything constantly changes and you must keep adjusting to stay balanced.

The Chinese sage Chuang Zi defined chi by saying, "Human life is a gathering of chi. If it disperses, one is no more."[8]

When a decision is made to try acupuncture, a number of questions are asked in order to define the problems. Everything that is felt or done or thought may be the root of disease. Practitioners will ask about exercise, diet, meditation, and philosophy of life. Anything can have an impact on a sense of well-being. All of it is involved with chi.

The client will then be asked to lie down on a table. The acupuncturist will place tiny steel needles at intervals along the energy pathways of his or her body. The needles, about the thickness of a human hair, do not hurt when inserted. Some people may find it a momentary discomfort, but others say they don't even know when the needle enters. Some acupuncturists twirl the needles. Others may use a little electricity. Still others use heat.

The acupuncturist verifies what is happening by checking the changes in pulse rate and any alterations in the color of skin tone. The goal of acupuncture is to help move from stillness to activity and back to stillness.

Moxibustion is another way to change and recharge chi. The moxa is made from finely ground mugwort leaves. It comes in the form of a cigarette or a small cone. The cigarette (or cone) is lit with a match, then placed on the acupuncture point and removed as soon as the patient feels it beginning to burn. Patients report that it feels warm and nourishing. The procedure usually does not even leave a blister. There is no danger of scarring.

If you want a clearer and more comprehensive picture of acupuncture treatment, J.R. Worsley has written a small book called, *Is Acupuncture for You?*[9] That may help you make up your mind.

Bob retained his sense of humor. He suggested to the acupuncturist that she might stimulate his face. He had heard about acupuncture facelifts and he figured he might as well emerge from his treatment looking younger. The acupuncturist said, "No problem."

The next week when he went in for his chemotherapy appointment, the receptionist and the other patients all commented that he looked quite fit. He chuckled and said, "Well, I don't know if the acupuncture helped, but it didn't hurt!"

In terms of why acupuncture has been so successful in the management of pain, studies done on rats show brains have specific receptors that react to stimulation. The scientists analyzed what happened when the rats' nerve centers were touched. The experiments showed that endorphins manufactured and multiplied in situ.

The endorphins acted as an analgesic. The brains manufactured their own opiates. This could explain why acupuncture works so well in calming the pain-alarm system.

Chinese Herbs

The Chinese have studied herbs for well over 5,000 years. They have organized and categorized thousands of herbs, placing them in three different groups: food, medicinal, and poisonous.

They have found that the food herbs nurture specific systems of the body by working directly on the digestive system. They aid our overall functioning.

The medicinal herbs act in the same way as Western drugs do. They control body functions, alleviate pain, and reduce swelling. Many of these medicinal herbs are ingredients used in Western drugs. The poisonous herbs can cause illness or death. Avoid them!

Nutrition

When you eat whole foods, you derive energy. Your body regenerates and functions in a healthier manner. The Chinese have long believed that your body has the ability to heal itself when fed properly.

Western medicine agrees that what you eat can help or hinder your well-being. As far back as 400 B.C., Hippocrates said, "Let food be your medicine and medicine be your food."[10] More and more physicians emphasize good nutrition. We now have low cholesterol diets, vegetarian diets, salt-free diets, and just plain sensible diets (low in fats and sugars). Changing your eating habits can make an enormous difference in dealing with any and all diseases.

Everyone knows that what you eat is important, but there have been so many fads and conflicting opinions that it can be difficult to decide what to do. Drink milk? Avoid all dairy? You need protein. You need fiber. Do you need carbohydrates? Avoid all meat, avoid only red meat, and avoid fish too? Everyone seems to have an opinion.

Starting at the beginning, the carbohydrates that you eat are broken down by your saliva into simple sugars. As the food is chewed and swallowed, it moves down through the digestive tract into the stomach. It then is transformed into enzymes and hydrochloric acid. After a time it moves to the small intestines, absorbing whatever nutrients are available along the way. Then it moves on into the colon, where it is transformed into waste product. The food provides the energy that enables us to walk and talk and think and breathe. If the food that is eaten is healthy, it will help form a protection against carcinogens and pollutants that are rampant throughout our environment. It will prevent the formation of unstable molecules. It will maintain strong bones. If you don't get enough vitamins and minerals, you won't have the ability to function properly. The problem is not if you should maintain a good diet, but how to choose which diet will do the most for you.

Poisons not to be put in our bodies include: alcohol, tobacco, caffeine, or other social drugs; unnecessary medications; food fried in oils, lard, or margarine; sugar, dextrose, corn syrup, saccharin, aspartame, or acesulfame-k; refined white flour; refined, over-processed, or synthetic food; artificial colors, sulfites, nitrates, BHA, BHT, and MSG.

Limit the following: animal proteins and fat such as beef, pork, dairy, and Bambi Burgers; salt (beware of pickled foods—olives, pickles, etc.); honey, maple syrup, and molasses; and fish, fowl, and eggs (buy organic).

Let's look at how to eat. Systematic undereating is an important nutritional tip for most people.

The diet should consist of substantial amounts of raw, whole, fresh, clean, nutrient, seasonal food.

Seventy-five percent of daily caloric intake should come from complex carbohydrates. Proteins should comprise fifteen percent and fats ten percent. A wise blend of whole grains, beans and seeds, legumes, and fresh vegetables should form the core of one's diet. This also assures high fiber.

Eat only when hungry.

Eat slowly in a relaxed and unhurried atmosphere. Eat several small meals rather than a few large meals.

Chew food well.

Never eat when in pain, mental or physical discomfort, or when working strenuously either physically or mentally.

Eat your last meal at least three or four hours before bedtime.

Drink plenty of pure water, particularly between meals. More is needed during lactation, exercise, and in the hot summer months. Soda, Kool-Aid, and other sugar-laden beverages are unacceptable.

Eat a diversity of foods.

It is best to rotate specific foods to once every two days.

Keep healthy snacks available, such as carrots, celery sticks, fruit, and rice cakes.

You might want to learn about the McDougall Program,[11] the Kempner[12] diet, which was developed at Duke University, the Pritikin[13] diet, or the diet recommended by Dean Ornish, M.D.[14] Some of the diets are more stringent than others. All have their proponents. Dr. Ornish is particularly concerned about and helpful for people who have heart disease. John McDougall, M.D., believes his diet helps with almost everything. Macrobiotic diets have been reported as useful to people with cancer.

Many people have also had good results with asparagus therapy.

Asparagus Therapy

Put canned asparagus into a blender. After blending, store in a glass jar in the refrigerator. Take four tablespoons morning and night.

Patients report feeling better in two to four weeks.

Take regularly for at least six months.

Fresh asparagus can be used but must be cooked.

For more information on this, write to International Association of Cancer Victims & Friends, P.O. Box 27387, Tucson, AZ 85726.

This short chapter can't thoroughly cover the large subject of nutrition. Please check out and explore further information with your physician or dietitian.

Biofeedback

In this age of understanding the mind-body connection, biofeedback training provides one means of gaining control of bodily processes. Through the use of computer technology, you learn how to control your physiological system. You can actually control blood flow, muscle activity, brain waves, temperature, sweat glands, heart rate, and breath rate.

It takes time and patience, but the results can be phenomenal. In the Biofeedback Training & Research Center in Cotati, California, Steven Wall has developed a program that he calls Biointegration.[15] He uses specialized instruments to monitor the body. Sensors placed on the forehead, shoulders, jaw, and scalp give signals that activate moving graphs on a computer screen. As you watch the muscle contractions on the screen, you become aware of how you are responding to tension.

Wall uses coordinating audio tones to help you let go. He has created computer patterns for you to color with your mind. As you quiet both your muscles and your brain, all sorts of things happen on the computer screen. The training process is challenging and fun.

It works with small children as well as adults. Biofeedback has taught youngsters to learn how to move different muscles, enabling them to walk when the regular system has been impaired. It has shown people how to relax their jaws so that TMJ and teeth grinding disappear. It has been helpful in cases of asthma and often reduces chronic pain.

Bob didn't try biofeedback, but I worked with a client who was in an automobile accident, which eventually resulted in Parkinson's disease. She had used traditional medicine, physical therapy, and chiropractic therapy, all of which helped a little. Still she experienced tremors and rigidity. Finally she embarked on biofeedback training. Through the training program, she developed the ability to sense when a tremor was about to break through. She noticed that when her mind remained calm, her body stayed quiet. She noticed different qualities in her tremors.

She said, "There is a tremor caused by anxiety, different from a tremor caused by lack of self-confidence or self-worth, different from the tremor that is caused by pain, and different from the tremor that the brain quietly allows because it feels normal. I can make a small mental adjustment and it is no longer there. The adjustment feels simple and direct. It is there in much the same way that lazy eyes cross when they are very tired. Somehow the brain muscle becomes tired and allows the tremor to soothe it. It takes a small effort to put it back on track. I can calm down at will."

Biofeedback is not a treatment, but rather an educational process for learning mind-body skills. This complementary path often provides relief from stress-related medical problems.

Massage and Aromatherapy

Many people find massage relaxing and comforting. Some physicians recommend it. Others caution against it in particular physical situations. Massage can be combined with aromatic oils and essences to encourage healing. There is an anecdote about a French cosmetic chemist, Rene-Maurice Gattefosse, Ph.D., who burned his hands from a laboratory explosion. Lavender essence helped stop the damage and began the healing.

Modern medicine accepts that some scents promote the healing of wounds. Physicians at Yale University and also the University of Pennsylvania are investigating the healing properties of garlic consumption. They think it may be helpful in reducing high blood pressure. New studies from Japan contend that oils from peppermint and cardamom can reduce spasms in the intestines.

When you decide to investigate a complementary approach, ask yourself the following nine questions.

Complementary Therapy Checklist

1. Does this therapy make any sense?
2. Does this therapy produce side effects?
3. Will I continue or stop the therapy based on my personal experience of it? Or will I allow myself to be influenced by other people? If so, why?
4. Will this treatment interfere in any way with my primary treatment?
5. Have I checked out the qualifications of the therapist?
6. Is there any validation that this treatment has been useful to others?
7. Do I have any or enough knowledge as to how and where this therapy originated?
8. What can and cannot be accomplished by undergoing this therapy?
9. Would there be value in discussing this treatment with my physician?

There are so many concepts floating around. A strong belief in the efficacy of a particular approach will make it work for you. I hope that, whatever you decide to do, you will do it with your eyes wide open. Keep your feet on the ground, a prayer in your heart, and a curious, adventurous attitude.

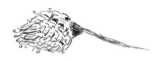

6

Family Reunion and the Social Atom

*Life is a great big canvas, and you should splash
all the paint on it that you can.*

Carole Rue, artist

We planned our summer family reunion with great care. Because Bob
needed to rest a great deal and because of our grandchildren's varied ages, we
decided that renting RVs would be a good solution.

Each family contingent would have its own space. It would be a great
adventure for all of us to camp as a caravan. So we sent out the invitations
and our seven sons and daughters-in-law responded with a resounding
unanimous yes.

Camp and swim meets were skipped. Vacations were rearranged. There
were fourteen adults and nine children, ranging in age from one to fourteen.
It took coordination and commitment, but every member of our big tribe

worked it out. Some of the family lives in the east, some in the west. Getting everyone together was a massive happening.

Two of us drove the RVs up to our property in shifts and parked the rigs in a circle. We were ready.

When the big day arrived, Bob couldn't get out of bed. He had developed a severe infection. Our carefully thought-out plans of camping under the stars and canoeing with the older boys couldn't happen. Instead Bob went to the hospital. His enormous disappointment added to his illness.

The RVs remained at the starting point and all the family adjusted to the situation. We grandparents had been so ready to focus outward on the next generation. But the situation turned inward. My top priority was Bob.

Each of the young families (usually concentrated on their individual family units) expanded their concern to include us. Our needs became theirs. They took over food preparations even as they devised treasure hunts to keep the small children occupied. They set up a volleyball net and took turns watching each other's children.

They scheduled visits to Bob in groups of twos and threes. What a gift. Something wonderful began to happen in the midst of disaster. We recognized we were a family!

The children understood it too. My granddaughter Zoë, six years old, chose a visit to the hospital to sing her Grandpa a lullaby instead of working on a jigsaw puzzle with her cousins.

At night we gathered in a circle and recounted old family stories. We laughed together and teased and created tighter bonds. In the morning those of us who were not visiting Bob danced the hokey pokey and threw water balloons.

As each team spent their hour with Bob, they let him know how much he meant to them. It was as healing as his medication.

Illness makes demands. Just as individuals go through developmental phases, so do the individual nuclear family units. At times, families are very close, very dependent on each other. If the illness is short-term, the family can usually manage it quite well. During a crisis period everyone wants to pitch in and the adrenaline runs on high. It can be a time of reaffirmation. We built some of our most beautiful memories during our reunion time.

We had planned to stay together a week and hoped every day that the hospital would release Bob. The doctor finally agreed he could come home Saturday. The easterners' return-trip tickets were for Sunday.

We decided to create an extraordinary homecoming for Bob. I called a rabbi friend of mine and asked if he would come to help Bob and me to renew our marital vows. He came with a portable bridal canopy. My friend Ruth agreed to sing. We assigned four of my grandchildren to hold the posts of the chupa.

Bob got into the spirit of it and, weak as he was, he put a tuxedo jacket over his pajamas and donned a top hat. We each wrote a vow and spoke them to each other through our tears. What a treasured memory for us all.

When family members have a common ground, they can work through any wrinkle that crops up. And they will crop up. How can we play volleyball when Dad is miserable? How can we be dancing the hokey pokey? Should we stay at the hospital full time? Am I giving more than you are?

Rabbi Hillel wrote, "If I am not for myself who will be for me? If I am only for myself what am I? If not now, when?"

At our reunion we struggled and talked about our feelings. We shared family memories and in the process made new ones.

Together we explored questions such as: Am I doing enough? Am I thinking only of myself? How and where is the balance? Most of us have a highly developed inner critic and have never learned how to be gentle with ourselves. Survivor guilt can often muddy relationships.

Researcher Lee Combrinck-Graham, Ph.D.,[16] sees the family system as a spiral that vibrates and moves between closeness and disengagement.

When a member of the family becomes ill, the illness changes all equations. As realization of the illness dawns, the family pulls inward. Energy concentrates on the illness. While some family members mobilize quickly, others take longer. This doesn't mean that anyone is dysfunctional or emotionally stuck. It is simply a matter of style.

We are all attached to the way things are. Whatever is familiar becomes a frame of reference. A change in vitality comes as a surprise. Those of us who are older are always a little bit shocked when we catch a glimpse of ourselves in the mirror. We expect to see the young person we were and know that he or she is in there somewhere, but where? We place an internal lock on the way we were. We don't release it easily.

Our economics, our intelligence, our appearance, whether we feel loved and respected, our sexuality, and even our politics forge our flexibility. So many variables influence the ways in which we cope with new challenges.

It is a good thing to remind ourselves that every ending leads to a new beginning. Every beginning eventually comes to an end. Every transition is affected by the ways in which we adapt to our culture, our race, our religion, and the people who live next door.

Adult development psychologist and author Daniel Levinson, Ph.D., says, "All transitions inherently involve the basic processes of termination and initiation. Arrivals and departures and losses are common life events, during which there is a preoccupation with death and finiteness."

The best way to approach any new situation is to acknowledge all the mixed feelings you have about it. As bad as a situation seems, you may find secondary gains inherent in it. Illness may bring relief from a boring job. You may discover a part of yourself that thoroughly enjoys fussing or being fussed over. The illness of your mate reaffirms that you are needed. A hundred million possibilities can influence your endurance and persistence.

It is normal to be affected by the timing and duration of the demands made on you. Take the time now to review how you have dealt with transitions in the past. Think back to all of the changes you have made. Do you become the comforter? Do you get anxious? Do you become directive under duress? How have you managed your behavior and brought it to a close?

For most people, acknowledging their grief brings relief. Many people find that they rethink the things most important to them.

Recognize that there is always a period of feeling cast adrift. After that period ends, you'll discover a chance to experience the "soul" part of every human experience. The literature of survivors repeatedly mentions spiritual awakening and deepening emotional bonds. You may find a golden nugget buried somewhere in the mud. We grow and learn in shadow as well as in light.

When an illness becomes chronic, the challenge becomes one of dealing with imposed restrictions. It is draining. Ongoing physical care requires alertness. Transitions that go on and on are harder on everyone.

When the disease is recurrent and has ups and downs, family members have a propensity toward burnout. It isn't unusual to get angry with the patient for disrupting your schedule. It isn't unusual for a patient to be angry with himself or herself for causing the disruption. Even when the patient is asymptomatic, the shadow of disease continues to haunt day-to-day activities.

Anticipation of further loss and/or untimely death is part of the state of flux. Each family has to figure out a way to develop breathing room. Under the stress of the moment, you may lose sight of the importance of taking time out to assess where and when and how to gather support.

Consider support groups as a resource. We know that families and friends want to help, but often they don't know how. Support group members have often told me that they feel much better after discussing their concerns in a place where others are considering similar problems.

Bob belonged to a men's group. When he became too ill to go to it, the men simply switched the meeting to our house. They would say to me as they arrived, "No women allowed. Come back in two hours." As Tiny Tim would say, "God bless them every one." Those men helped me retain my sanity.

At some point, we had to consider hospice. So will you. For many of us, making that call is the recognition that death is imminent. We may try to push the realization away, not realizing what a relief hospice care offers.

Originally a hospice was a way station for pilgrims and tired travelers, a place to rest, refresh, and often share stories of the adventure. It still is, although now hospice care is usually administered in one's own home, a family member's home, or in a nursing home.

The word hospice comes from Latin and means guesthouse or resting spot. Today it has come to mean palliative care. The new concept of hospice started in London at St. Christopher's Hospital in the 1960s as the vision of Dame Cicely Saunders, M.D., who believed that people had the right to die with dignity and without pain. The first hospice in the United States was established in New Haven, Connecticut, in 1974.

Hospice neither ends nor extends life. It utilizes caregivers, nurses, physicians, and volunteers to enrich the lives of terminal patients with tender loving care.

Death is a natural process all too often seen as a battle. Hospice workers learn ways to ease the process. They use physical and occupational therapists to help patients cope with disability. They use social workers to help patients express feelings and mediate family conflicts. They help patients negotiate systems. Physicians and nurses utilize the latest pain management techniques and address all symptoms of the disease.

There are now more than 3,100 hospice programs in the U.S. Rather than a place, it is a protocol, a way of caring for a terminally ill patient at home, in the home of a family member, or in a nursing home. Physicians usually refer patients to hospice when they believe the patients are in the last six months of life.

Hospice workers train the primary caregiver (who may be a life partner, relative, or friend) to work closely with the professional staff. They show caregivers ways to bathe, turn, administer medications, and monitor changes in the patient's condition.

All hospice staff members are taught how to deal with the loneliness and fear often experienced by the patient and his or her loved ones. They work together with the primary caregivers to develop a personalized care plan. Pain and comfort levels, support systems, financial and insurance resources, medications, and equipment needs are carefully evaluated.

Medicare covers the cost of hospice care for patients with a prognosis of six months or less, but a patient can remain in hospice care beyond six months if the physician recertifies the illness as terminal.

Benefits cover all services related to the illness including physician services; nursing and home health aids; medical appliances and supplies; dietary counseling; continuous care during crisis periods; trained volunteers; and bereavement services.

Hospice staff is on call twenty-four hours a day, seven days a week. If you want to locate a hospice near you, check the Yellow Pages under "Hospice" or call the Hospice Foundation of America at 1-800-854-3402 and ask for an admissions representative.

When I first mentioned hospice to Bob, he brushed me off by saying, "I don't need that."

I said simply, "I do." Finally, I talked him into accepting the idea of "pre-hospice care." Our hospice folks came to the house and gently explained the program. He became comfortable with it and with them. He also let them know he only allowed them to come in order to help me.

It may still be too early for hospice in your case. But, even with all the help hospice can give, both patient and caregiver need additional support systems. To help you identify your possible aid stations, I have included two sociometric exercises. In one you can identify people who may be available or people who would be available with a small amount of reparative relationship work. This is for your own information, but it may be even more helpful if you share and discuss your findings with your partner. Use the exercises in a way that feels constructive and comfortable to you.

J.L. Moreno, M.D., known as the father of psychodrama, coined the term "social atom" in 1934. He designed it as a way of identifying your role relationships. Ann Hale has refined it and now uses a traffic light system to describe the kind of relationship you have with the people in your social atom.[18]

Green light is obviously a relationship with a positive flow of current.

Yellow is one with the caution light flashing. As you identify your interactions, you may want to spend a few minutes on figuring out what that cautionary note is about and what you can do to move it into a green connection.

Red relationships offer clues about when and where you have difficulty.

Jot them all down. Don't be polite. They will give you information on what you need to avoid or what sorts of behavior trap you into discomfort.

Personal Atom: Moreno's Social Atom
Nucleus of Persons Emotionally Related to You

Exploring Your Social Atom to
Develop a Support System that Works

1. Make a list of the friends and family members you are emotionally involved with.

2. Make a list of people with whom you would like to have a relationship.

3. Make a list of your acquaintances. I have a colleague, Ro King, who coined the term "amiary" to denote those people you really enjoy but don't see on a continual basis.

4. List them all. Include anyone and everyone who comes to mind. Don't edit.

5. Take a sheet of paper and place yourself in the center. Use a circle to symbolize women and a triangle for the men in your life. Place them on the graph according to how close or distant they feel to you.

6. If they are green lights (positive), use a green line to connect them to you.

7. If they are yellow (neutral), use a yellow line.

8. If they are red (troublesome relationship), use a red line.[19]

Stay aware of what you feel as you do this. When you finish, you might want to check out whether the "red" folks have anything in common.

Community Atom: Social Atom Collectives Exploration

1. Make a list of groups that mean something to you. List them even if you are not active in them anymore. You may want to jot down groups you would wish to join. Don't limit yourself.
2. Take a sheet of paper and put yourself in the middle of it. Name each group and draw a circle on the page to represent that group's importance. Use the size of the circle to indicate how important that group is to you and draw lines between you and the group to indicate what you feel about the group just as you did with your personal atom.
   - Green line means you are positively attracted.
   - Yellow line means you are neutral about it.
   - Red line means you are repelled by the group.

Consider groups such as family, friends, work, church, medical helpers, support groups, hospital, hospice, Cancer Society, Lupus Society, and so on.

Number the groups in order of their importance to you in your life, here and now. Include names of people who belong to a particular group.

Check to see if people appear in more than one of the groups. Identify the reason that group is important to you.[20]

Spend some time analyzing your findings. Then choose an action that you would consider making so as to make your relationships greener. If you find that you have any reservation about taking an action, or if it doesn't seem right to you, ask yourself how come? What would make it easier? What do you need to make this good action happen for you? Let the answer come without judging yourself. If you encounter your "inner critic," tell him or her to get lost. You really know what is best for you to do. Trust yourself to do it. Do it now.

7

A Shadow in the Life Cycle and a Change in Activity

I believe there is another way of looking at life that makes it possible for us to walk through this world in love, at peace, and without fear. This other way requires no external battles, but only that we heal ourselves. It is a process I call "Attitudinal Healing," because it is an internal and primarily mental process. Properly practiced, it will, I believe, allow anyone, regardless of his or her circumstances, to begin to experience the joy and harmony that each instant contains, and to start his journey on a path of love and hope.

Gerald G. Jampolsky, M.D.

There is a time of recognition when you discover that your life isn't the way you thought it was going to be. Just as you begin to adjust to one loss, another one comes along. Sometimes you share your sadness with your partner and sometimes you don't.

In the process, you find a sense of heightened appreciation for little things like sharing the Sunday newspaper and feeling the warmth of an arm around you as you cuddle up and watch a video.

It was a time for holding on and letting go. Bob was tired. I came home in the early evening and found him lying down for a nap. His rhythm was changing. He never went to his meeting of independent investors. Instead, he curled up with a book and didn't get dressed all day. I felt the stab of panic in my diaphragm but I made light of it. If that is what felt good to him, it should be fine with me.

I'd seen a big shift in his behavior patterns. He had always been full of bravado. He had always pushed himself to the limit. Nothing was ever a problem. We all know that we must deal with death at some point in our journey. But when a serious diagnosis has been given, we feel the imperative to plan, to talk, to be in this together.

Bob's fatigue set off a small alarm. It hinted that there would be an ending at some point in the future. I wanted to believe his fatigue was transient and unimportant. I wanted to view it as an opportunity for discussion, as a push toward honest appraisal for him, a pull for me to be self-reliant, and nothing more. It didn't feel like that. It scared me. It frightened him too. We would force ourselves not to ignore it.

I knew I could hike up the hills alone, travel alone, go to the movies alone. But I didn't want to. I didn't want to think about doing anything alone. One day I went to visit my grandson and made a wrong turn on a road I knew well. I had taken this route a hundred times before, but I was not paying attention. I was alone in my car, aware of my aloneness. I got lost.

I didn't want to accept any alteration in Bob's and my relationship. I rationalized and reframed that his tiredness was just one of those things. I made myself believe that tomorrow all would be just as it was yesterday. We both knew we should discuss what was going on, but we pretended once more that nothing was amiss. Most of us do not know how to handle loss. I was no exception. I resisted changes and avoided endings.

Bob didn't like it when pain medication made him groggy, so he put off taking it as long as he could. He knew that he wasn't as strong and alert as he had been, but he believed that admitting to discomfort would make it a reality. He resisted as hard and as long as he could.

I knew that he was hurting but I didn't want to address the problem. We both skirted the issue. His growing-up myth was that it was important to keep fear and sadness to oneself. If he acknowledged what he felt, then he would have to do something about it. He knew that the only thing he could do was to accept these changes, but he simply refused to do that.

Bob kept his fast pace up until the day he found himself gripping the wheel to stay awake and in control. Then he pulled over to the side of the road and called me to come pick him up. He finally acknowledged that he could cause an accident. He had to let go of his pride so he wouldn't be a danger on the road. He entered into this more restricted phase of life kicking and screaming, but he had courage. He always said that courage was when you are fearful but you do what you have to do anyway.

I let out a sigh of relief. I had been stuffing my worry for weeks. "I'll take you wherever you want to go," I said.

"I know," Bob answered, "but there will be times when we both resent my dependence. It's going to be hard for both of us."

"We can talk it through," I said.

"I feel helpless," he said.

"I know," I answered. It was a breakthrough.

John James, the founder of the Grief Recovery Institute, located in Sherman Oaks, California, and Ontario, Canada, says there are five stages of grieving that have to be addressed each and every time loss is experienced.

1. Gaining awareness
2. Accepting responsibility
3. Identifying recovery communications
4. Taking actions
5. Moving beyond loss

Our experiences along life's road condition the way we respond to the current loss. We repeat the behaviors we have learned before, sometimes expanding on them, but more often responding in the same habitual rigid manner again and again. Whatever we did before seems familiar and easier to do than something new. We operate on automatic pilot. Conscious change takes grit.

If you want to find another way of responding, try doing the following exercise. It will work better if your partner participates with you, but you can gain understanding even if you do it on your own.

Developing a Loss Graph

Draw a line to represent your life. Begin with your birth at one end and your death at the other.

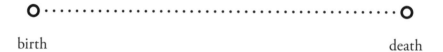

birth   death

Where are you now on your journey? Place a mark on that place. It may be halfway or three quarters of the way, or almost at the very end. Don't think about it; just let your intuition guide you to the place on the graph that seems most accurate.

Now make as many marks as you need along your lifeline to indicate losses that are significant to you. They may be big or small. Don't judge; just let whatever comes to mind out on the paper. Label the losses. It may be the time Mom gave away your cat, or the time you couldn't go away to camp because money was tight, or when Grandfather died. Loss comes in many guises.

Now look at what you jotted down on your line.

What was it that you learned with each loss?

Did you pick up the idea that you shouldn't cry?

That you should grieve by yourself?

That you should always put on a happy face? That you can make the loss better by getting another dog or buying a new bike?

Perhaps you learned you shouldn't trust people, or that you need to protect yourself at all times.

Maybe you found out it is important not to think about your loss or that the quicker you distract yourself the better.

Make a note of the injunctions that came up for you and ask your partner to do the same for his or hers.

The losses may be big or little and some may stir up uncomfortable old feelings. When you have finished your graph and thought about it, share it with your partner. This is an opportunity to discover the ways in which each of you have dealt with your losses. It can make a difference in how you both face the events in your lives right now. Start with one loss and explore your reaction and the messages you received from your family and friends about that loss.

Take as much time as you need and listen to each other without interruption.

When the time came for Bob to stop driving, he freed up space in his life. His first reaction was to be disoriented and sometimes demanding. Then, because he had always been pragmatic and curious, he began to explore his situation. He had to accept his new boundaries and set a new pattern for his existence. He then had time to read and think. He watched a pair of robins nest and saw when the fledglings began to fly. He noticed the banana slugs in the garden and marveled at their ugliness. He did less. He observed more.

Psychologist Stanley Keleman writes, "Life can be described as a migration through many formative loops, many little dyings. Growth, change and maturing occur by deforming the old and forming the new. In the little dyings we can learn how to live our big dying. [21]

There was a parallel change in me as well. We spent one afternoon looking at family photographs. I found a snapshot of my oldest son skipping stones, then another of my second son on his first two-wheeler bike. He looked so proud. I recalled the persistence it took for him to achieve balance. We chuckled together. It was a good day.

That led to the photograph of Bob at college. We stared at a picture of the old high school gang bundled up in down coats, standing on their ice skates amid tall weeds that stubbornly resisted the winter ice.

"Memories do go on," I thought. "Change is natural. I'm not that teenager anymore. My grandson is the teenager now." We both took a small step toward accepting death. We began to categorize what was important and what was not. We decided to write that down.

Many generations ago, it was a Jewish tradition to write an ethical will and put it into the care of the rabbi to read after the funeral.

An ethical will is a document distinctly different from a property will. It doesn't concern who inherits what. Rather, it involves observations and desires that the writer would like to have his or her survivors consider. It is an acknowledgment that while society will go on without his or her physical presence, some people can carry on his or her ideas. The ethical will gives you the opportunity to have your say. You might want to write your own. You'll find it a fine opportunity to review and evaluate your meaningful experiences.

Bob's Ethical Will

Dear Family:

I can't remember a single incident or story that I feel I must pass on to you but I want you to know that I have worked hard in the last few years in our temple and I have searched for harmony and tranquility. I don't know why but I have never had a particular objective. I've just done it.

My life has been good and full, enriched by Maryann and each of you, my family.

I want you to know how much I love you and how glad I am that you have been my family and my teachers.

I wish that each of your lives exceed your expectations. Mine has.

I never felt the need to acknowledge my endeavors but I have enjoyed them... especially swimming naked in the Housatonic River.

It is important for me to be my own person, carry my own identity—I hope you will do the same. Whatever works for you.

I have always had difficulty in expressing myself but I hope you know how much I cared for each of you.

My only regret is that I haven't been sensitive to your needs.

You are bringing up your children in a totally different way and haven't repeated my errors and I am pleased about that. Every generation is a different generation faced with new challenges.

I cannot define true success—here again it is up to you but whatever that is, I want it for you.

I hope that I have made a difference for having been here and that you will remember me without frills.

Your Dad

Bob Schacht

My Ethical Will

I, Maryann Schacht, being of sound mind and full heart do leave to you my family and friends and all fellow human beings all these things which I believe have been most important to me on my life journey. These are the lessons of my lifetime.

Listen to the bird song and notice the yellow mustard fields in spring.

In summer, head down to the lake and jump in, preferably without clothes. Listen to the gurgle of water as your arms pull you through the lake. It is wonderful to cut through the water's skin. It resists gently. It holds you in the same caress as amniotic fluid. I believe that death is like that too. I am not afraid of floating.

When Indian summer comes gather cherries in the red gold warmth of the clear harvest day. Climb as high into the tree as you can and look out from your perch as far as you can. Eat some of the cherries before you descend and let the juice drip down your chin.

Take a walk in the winter snow. Build a snowman. Slide down the hill on a cardboard box lid. I never melted although my toes felt frozen and it was always worth it to come home to hot chocolate and oatmeal cookies.

If you do catch a cold, curl up under a soft down quilt and pamper yourself. The world will go on. Chores can wait.

Make the time to play with the children. Get to know them. They grow up so fast. I have so loved being a mother. It has been the best achievement of all.

Any time of year ride out over the countryside on a Peruvian Paso mare. That is living!

The most charming moments are stretching ones, the daring ones. I have loved the friskiness of my small risks.

It is important to leave this world a little changed for the better. I don't know that I have accomplished that but I have tried. Actually the trying has been everything from aggravating to exhilarating.

Remember birthdays and share earnest conversations and special meals with lovers and friends and children. Those are the best of times.

Pet and please the animals. Those that have come to live with me have all given me so much joy (not always unadulterated).

There was a resident herd of deer that never learned they weren't supposed to eat the vinca vines, and dogs that have chewed a hole in the bedroom carpet, and the cat that ate our Thanksgiving turkey. Those have become cherished memories.

What I have learned is that you just don't know. Expect to be surprised and never get over being astonished.

It is important to remember that we are only one of many species that share this earth. It is not ours alone.

I have husbanded my small corner of this universe so full of strange grasses and colorful flowers.

Take the opportunity to savor all its variety, all its gardens, both cultivated and wild.

As a reminder I have bought packets of poppy seeds and wildflowers for you to scatter wildly or plant in good earth and water conscientiously. This world so needs its plants and trees. Take up my job, pick up my shovel and use my rake. Be stewards of the planet.

Listen. I want to share a secret. There are storytellers here and everywhere. Each has a story to tell and if you listen well, you learn and grow in spirit.

Read history. It keeps repeating. If each one of us reads about the past we may just change the future.

Ease up. Slow down. Out the door is not better. I have enjoyed this past year. Ordinary tasks are or can be pathways of meditation. Ironing a tablecloth can be time out for contemplation. Deliberate daily chores can quiet the chatter in your head. Do the dishes and walk the dog, and recycle the garbage without resentment.

I leave you the enchantment of complexity. Paradox may be troubling but it stops you from taking anything for granted.

I bequeath you care and concern for yourself and for each other. I encourage you to discover your own way of unfolding and accept it joyfully. I leave you an affirmation badge that says "I Am Unique" because you are.

Maryann Schacht

Life isn't always the way you want it to be. It has a beginning, a middle, and an end. All of it changes. We have to change with it. We have no choice about that.

It is difficult to think about a funeral, yet throughout our lives we mark our special occasions with rites of passage: birth, graduation, marriage, sometimes divorce, and eventually death.

We send cards and flowers and gather together with friends and family. Ceremony is a phenomenon that transcends all cultures and survives throughout human history.

Why? Are rites of passage really necessary?

Ritual, though certainly not required, seems to help us move from what was to what will be. Ritual soothes our fear during the upheaval of transition. Ritual becomes an outlet that channels the excitation that moves arm in arm with disruption. Only when we allow ourselves to fully experience the disorientation of change can we move past the discomfort and find a true sense of resolution.

The funeral ritual helps put a period at the end of the sentence. It allows the mourners the chance to begin to work through their denial and anger to express their sadness and to do something meaningful. Gathering for a goodbye makes the death real. Having friends around affirms that the survivor is not alone.

Some people think that they are sparing their family by asking that no one take notice of their death, but it actually makes the grieving process more difficult. Grief can become pathological when the survivor refuses to let go.

There are a variety of approaches and many ways to say farewell. You might want to put some effort into deciding what kind of ceremony would be best for you now, while you are in a position to be in charge.

Some religions have prescribed formal ceremonies. Some are less formal. Some people write their own memorials, choose the hymns they want sung and the refreshments that they want served. Others would rather leave all the arrangements up to their significant other. Think it over. Talk it through.

People can meet on a golf course as well as in a church. Jim Henson, the creator of the Muppets, wanted a parade at his funeral. He wanted his memorial service to be joyous, and it was. He created a celebration that was held in the Church of St. John the Divine in New York City. His Muppets were there, and a band played. It was a celebration.

One of my clients had a farewell party while he was still alive to enjoy it. He planned and attended his own wake. He sipped champagne with his friends and said his goodbyes with tears and laughter and died the next morning.

The sort of ceremony that is arranged is not as important as the fact that a particular life is acknowledged. When you know that your life has made a difference to many people, it isn't polite to disappear without leaving a trace.

Consider that children and grandchildren do much better psychologically when they are included. Remember your loss graph and what it tells you about building in responses?

Did you know that within hours after death the surviving partner has to make at least fifty separate and urgent decisions? He or she has to notify the doctor or coroner and get in touch with the funeral director and the cemetery or memorial park. He or she then has to contact relatives and friends, arrange for a minister or speaker. If one has been working, an employer needs to be advised. Someone needs to write an obituary. A casket or urn or small plain box may have to be selected. Clothing for the funeral needs to be chosen, flowers ordered, music selected, food arranged, and transportation managed. The surviving partner will want to acknowledge notes of sympathy with printed stationery, a card, or a letter. Inevitably the bills will come in and they have to be paid. There is so much to be done at the time when the survivor is least capable of thinking in an organized way. Having advance directives makes it manageable.

Writing instructions down in advance helps ensure that everything will be done the way the patient wished.

As difficult as it may seem, the finest gift a patient can give a caregiver is to consider the following questions in advance.

Do you want to be buried or cremated?

Where do you want to be buried or cremated?

If a burial were your choice, what kind of casket would you prefer?

Do you want to leave a photograph or suggestions for how you want your hair fixed, and what you want to wear?

Where do you want your service held? Who will officiate?

Do you have a special charity you want mentioned so that people can make donations in your name?

Is there a special poem you want read?

Do you want a particular piece of music played?

You might even consider writing your own obituary. How would you like to be remembered? Perhaps the two of you might write your thoughts down together. It is just fine to make up your own exit.

A Guide To Help Organize Your Information.

Name of mortuary _____

Name of deceased _____

Address _____

Birthplace _____

Date and place of death _____

Schools attended _____

Degrees and affiliations _____

Occupation or when retired from where _____

Previous or other occupations _____

Club, professional, church affiliations and offices held _____

_____

Other information of interest, such as pioneer family? _____

_____

Local history or special activities or services _____

Survivors and cities where they reside:

Spouse or life companion _____

Parents _____

Daughters _____

Sons _____

Sisters _____

Brothers _____

Grandchildren _____

Great grandchildren _____

Friends may call (time and place) _____

Or wake and rosary (time and place) _____

Funeral services (time and place) _____

Or Requiem mass (time and place) _____

Officiating clergy or other _____

Where burial or entombment or cremation_____

Pallbearers _____

Honorary bearers _____

Donations to _____

Life is precious and holding on to it as long as we can is highly valued by our society, but there is a time when dying becomes the preferred choice.

My friend Sister Marietta fought long and hard until she came to the place where she accepted that letting go was God's will. She told me she would like to die on a saint's day and she did. She held out until her name day. When that day arrived, she closed her eyes and breathed her last. Accepting that dying is a natural process allows it to be just that. It is when we jettison our fear and accept the totality of life that we achieve a good death.

The temple bell stops
But the sound keeps coming out of the flowers.

Basho

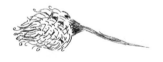

8

Wedding Rings and Expectations

Oft expectation fails, and most oft there
Where most it promises.

William Shakespeare

My wedding ring was tight. I tried turning it, but my finger was too swollen. It wouldn't budge. I was stubborn; my sheer determination moved it ever so slightly. Then pop—it bounced on the floor. I panicked, frightened it was gone forever. Then I saw it a foot away, melting into the design of the Oriental carpet. My finger looked so empty. I felt as though I had just ended my marriage.

I didn't want Bob to see that my ring was gone. I didn't want Bob to think that I had given up on us. I didn't want him to see my bare finger. I had to get my ring adjusted right away. I ran directly to the garage, got in my car, and hightailed it to the nearest jewelry store. Many customers waited in this mall store. Finally, the salesman nodded to me.

"How soon can you enlarge my ring?" I asked.

"It will take a week," he answered.

"It can't take a week. It just can't. We may not have a week!" I started to cry. The poor jeweler didn't know what to do. He had no way to cope with the emotional basket case unraveling in front of him. He tried to calm me down. I kept crying. It didn't matter that people were staring. Nothing mattered to me except getting my ring back on my finger.

At that moment the woman who actually did the ring sizing appeared and said, "This seems to be extremely important to you."

I almost remarked on her perceptiveness. Instead, I bit my tongue and said, "Yes."

"Look, how about if I have it back in two days?" I calmed down and settled for that offer. All the way home I kept rubbing my finger, looking for my wedding ring.

I hoped Bob wouldn't notice and yet I knew he would. I needed to tell him how much he meant to me. I needed to let him know that a wedding ring is only the outward sign of commitment. I needed to tell myself that too. We just might use this as an opportunity to talk. What is marriage, after all?

We live in a time when the media has deluged most of us with ideas about how we ought to be and how our relationships ought to be. Life partners are supposed to be friends, providers, lovers, islands of safety, and supportive mentors. Partners are supposed to intuit how we feel and agree with what we think. We expect our partners to replicate all of the good qualities that we found in our families of origin and also make up for all of our families' deficiencies.

We would be just fine if only our partners would be all of those things and do all of that. The trouble is that they can't and they don't. Relationships can only go so far. What they can do is create the opportunity to learn more about our self and more about someone else's self. Both members of the couple grow in the unfolding.

Life is all about learning how to be responsible for oneself while still contributing to the coupling. Pop psychology grinds out marvelous advice. It reminds us how often we set up unrealistic expectations of our significant others as well as of ourselves.

Our partners cannot know what is going on inside our heads. No one conceptualizes in the same way as another. Each one of us has his or her own unique life perspective.

My husband was a problem-solver. He addressed the task at hand. He was a "just-the-facts" kind of guy. I looked for the feeling tones. I dramatized. He didn't. It wouldn't occur to him to think that I might be trapped in a mind mudslide.

I agonized over the loss of his chest hair. He couldn't have cared less about that. He was preoccupied with gathering statistics on the next medical approach to undertake.

He lost his libido during the course of treatment. We both recognized it. We both agonized over our disappearing sex life. He could no longer sustain an erection. That impacted both of us but we didn't discuss it. In his attempt to spare me we were tiptoeing around each other. We kept trying to avoid our reality.

He cared about me, about himself, about us. I loved this man. I hated that he was hurting and I hated that I was hurting. I connected the dots realizing that these thoughts were directly connected to taking off my wedding ring.

I made up my mind. We had to confront our issue. We had to be absolutely honest with each other. If I talked about my sadness, he would be able to express his. We could respond to each other's pain and handle it. Our divergent perspectives would bring us closer.

I needed to find my courage and trust our relationship. Whenever we stopped our communication process, we retreated into isolation. As we heard each other, emotions began to shift.

We needed to address our concern about our loss of sexual connection. It was a reality that wouldn't disappear. Bringing it to the surface did not ordain devastation. We were always stronger when we solved problems together.

I was Bob's wife in sickness and in health, with or without a ring on my finger. We could still make love, with or without an erection. Orgasm could be achieved with a vibrator or a gentle touch.

The benefit of a good relationship is that one and one adds up to three: you, me, and that wonderful something that we share between us. Two heads are better than one when they cooperate with each other. As each contributes, the relationship becomes stronger and more resilient.

Because Bob was typically macho and stoic, he always found adjusting to any change difficult. He fought using a La-Z-Boy chair that could assist him in getting to his feet. He fought using a walker. He refused a wheelchair. He balked at the hospital bed.

I remember one time when we flew to Seattle for treatment. He created a scene at the airport. He barked at me, "I don't need a wheelchair. I am not a baby."

It took a good deal of patience and lots of placating. And to think my middle name is Impatience. I was grateful I had a hospice counselor available as a coach. Those weekly meetings helped me stay steady. My man was from time to time irascible!

"He doesn't mean it. It is not me. It's the illness," became my mantra. I often had to remind myself that this was the man I loved. I learned to monitor my own behavior and sometimes I slipped and snapped. There were times when I felt that both of us were dying and I wished for the end to come swiftly.

I took breaks, went for walks, and arranged for friends to drop in. After a movie I found I could deal in a more productive manner. We all need breaks.

Bob and I began to learn how to accept our humanity and especially our frailties. We talked our way through our blow-ups. We talked to each other after the explosions died down. We let each other know it was OK to let off steam. We acknowledged that we were living in a pressure cooker and that we were doing the best we could. We loved each other through the awful days and sleepless nights, and we forgave each other. More importantly, we accepted and forgave ourselves. Everyone responds to stress differently.

Some of us have anxious thoughts. We ruminate. We forget things. We find it hard to concentrate. These are cognitive symptoms.

Behavioral symptoms might include insomnia, tremors, crying, or a change in eating or drinking regimen. Emotionally, we may become irritable, restless, or depressed. Physiologically, we may grind our teeth, clench our fists, sweat, lose our sex drive, get a lump in our throat, or we may even become nauseated. We run to the bathroom or become constipated. We put on weight or lose weight. The list goes on and on.

On the social plane, we may find ourselves talking too much or avoiding contact. Daniel Goleman, Ph.D., and Joe Gurney, Ph.D., in collaboration with James Pennebaker at Southern Methodist University in Dallas, Texas, found that sharing feelings had a direct impact on the immune system. They assigned twenty-five students to keep journals in which they were asked to address personal and traumatic events in their lives. They gave a control group of twenty-five students topics that were lightweight in tone (e.g., descriptions of shoes or a social event). The other students were assigned heavy subjects.

After six weeks, laboratory tests on the participants' white blood cells were conducted. The students with serious subjects to discuss showed more activity and reactivity to mitogens, protein compliments found on the human genome. The health clinic reported that these students had had fewer illnesses and visited health centers less often. Their immune systems had become more active! Since there were no reported differences between the groups of students before the study began, the conclusion could be drawn that the differences were related to their expressive outlets.

Aside from the emotional closeness that occurs when we talk to each other, we benefit individually on a physiological level. Bottled-up thoughts add to stress and impact the body's ability to fight the assault of disease. It takes courage to express what one is thinking and feeling. Each partner has a tendency to protect the other and the desire to make everything easier for the other, but the evidence shows that a healing happens when a couple trusts enough to discuss the shadows—fear, a sense of vulnerability, and anger.

The first step is always the hardest. It feels like such a big risk.

Some couples can talk about concrete issues like what needs to be done and how to go about doing it. However, they may be closed on a particular subject such as Joe's procrastination at work or Mary's habit of talking for hours on the telephone. Whenever they touch on one of those toxic subjects, it ends in Sturm und Drang. The partners become critical and judgmental when they approach difficult topics. While each believes he or she is being open, the emotional connection is actually shutting down.

What will Joe think if Mary says she is terrified of what lies ahead? She projects that he will consider her a wimp. She worries that he doesn't love her enough to accept her timidity. She is convinced that she has to be stoic at all times to retain his admiration. Her squeamishness may come from the years she spent watching her mother deal with her father's diabetes. Her terror of needles may have everything or nothing to do with Joe. Now faced with the possibility of administering insulin medication, she finds herself tied up in knots.

Can they begin to talk about alternatives on an informational level? That is a starting place. It may be that having a visiting nurse administer the shot is a fine solution, or that Joe could do his own shots. Perhaps Mary will find her fear of needles dissipating after she watches once or twice.

This outcome would be fine. However, it still leaves Mary's fear of abandonment, her idea that he will leave if she doesn't measure up to his expectation, untouched. The best way to get past the dark place is to go into it. The longer one avoids dealing with a problem, the more the stress increases. It takes determination and courage and work to attain openness. The best way to approach is with tenderness. Mary needs to accept her underlying fear before she can modify it. Once she knows what she is dealing with, she can explain it to Joe.

If you find so much stress built up in your relationship that you are frozen or furious, relationship problems probably predate this stress.

Illness is a shock wave that triggers high anxiety and emotional arousal. It highlights whatever vulnerabilities already exist. It sets off reactivity and automatic responses. Partners find themselves craving attention and falling back into the unspoken expectations that each brought to the relationship when they entered into it. Some of those expectations may have been submerged or reluctantly put aside. Now that there is a threat to the marriage's stability, the safety factor changes.

In the midst of this new threat, what may have been relaxed becomes an area of tension. The four charged areas in a marriage are money, sex, parenting, and death. The first two issues, money and sex, relate to power. Parenting relates to influence. Death involves relinquishing both power and influence. Avoiding discussion is common, especially when we are competitive with one another. When a marriage works, power and influence are distributed in a fairly equal way. When a marriage is dysfunctional, both partners are out of balance. To achieve equality means risking self-disclosure and investing in open discussion. Sweeping feelings under the rug takes energy. It rarely works.

We all have the ability to read facial expressions and observe body language. Sighs and grimaces speak volumes. When couples live together they heighten their "meta" communication skills. They know on an instinctual level what is permissible and what is not. The unwritten contract keeps the relationship on an even keel by incorporating the defenses and myths of both partners. Each couple works out their own guidelines and sets their personal boundaries.

Ideally, each partner operates as a whole and separate person. The family therapists talk of being "differentiated." If we have solved the tasks of our development well enough in the early years, we know the difference between what we think and what we feel. We know the boundaries between others and ourselves.

Trouble develops if we use our mate to build our own self-esteem, as an antidote to anxiety, or to lift depression. When your partner is emotionally down, you must remain separate enough to carry on. We must not be fused to our mates. Your loved one should not be seen as an extension of yourself. We may be sad and certainly concerned but must still be able to stay within our own skin. It is important to let the physically challenged partner make decisions about treatment for himself or herself. Suggestions and discussion only help as long as we do not become coercive. It is hard, but we need to honor the patient's right to choose his or her own path.

If discussing your needs and thoughts with your partner feels too overwhelming at the moment, consider joining a support group for a safe place to explore what stops you from expression within your relationship. No marriage is perfect, but some have more impediments than others. In a support group, you will find that you are not alone. Everyone there is wrestling with similar issues and circumstances.

Some support groups are designed to encourage the expression of strong emotion. Pain, fear, anxiety, and wishful desires are all fair game. You can delve into any and all of them without worrying about being "judged." Once you do, it will become easier to be open within your family.

If you are the patient, you may be able to restructure your view by reframing your illness into a challenge. Others in the group will share tips on how to make your life more comfortable, ways in which they have learned to deal with fatigue or pain. As one of my clients said, "The group is the place to learn how to not sweat the small stuff." We can learn so much from one another. Start your search for a support group by asking your doctor, nurse, or social worker. Ask because many busy medical people forget to mention social support.

One of my clients had a lumpectomy. When she told her physician that she had finally found a group, he was surprised. He said, "You only had a lumpectomy." She responded, "If you lost a piece of your penis, you wouldn't think it was such a small thing!"

Though times are changing, you still have to ask for what you want. Organizations such as the American Cancer Society, the American Diabetes Association, or the American Heart Association often offer groups at little or no charge. If you belong to an HMO, you can inquire about support group availability through them. If you don't find anything available, consider enlisting help and starting one.

Not all support groups are the same. You certainly don't need to be in one that will add to your stress. Try the group out. If you come out of it feeling better than when you went in, that is a good sign. It may be that the discussion upsets you, but you still realize that you are always acquiring new knowledge. Try not to quit too soon. However, if you find you're bored or feel belittled, trust your instinct and look for a different group. There are also many groups for caregivers. Remember that the caregiver needs social support as much as the patient does. You are both under severe pressure. When you take care of yourself, it helps everyone concerned.

Your expectations have a great deal to do with the course and management of the disease. If you have the expectation that you can always grow and use every day as an opportunity to become more of who you really are, you will find that you have more energy available to manage the disease.

Researchers have found self-reliance and assertiveness to be two qualities that accompany spontaneous remission and longer survival. Holistic nurse and author Jeanne Achtenberg, Ph.D., found flexibility, insight, high ego strength, and the refusal to give up helped people in her study outlive their diagnoses.

If either of you have not tapped into your particular strengths yet, it isn't too late. Assertiveness, resourcefulness, and optimism can be learned. You can develop a nurturing, hopeful atmosphere with a little practice.

Guide to Relationship Openness

1. How would you rate yourself in terms of openness?
   Always   Mostly   Sometimes   Rarely   Never

2. Do you limit yourself to information or are you able to discuss your wants and feelings?
   Always   Mostly   Sometimes   Rarely   Never

3. Is your interchange critical?
   Always   Mostly   Sometimes   Rarely   Never

4. Is your interchange affectionate?
   Always   Mostly   Sometimes   Rarely   Never

5. Does your conversation indicate respect for your partner?
   Always   Mostly   Sometimes   Rarely   Never

6. Do you trust your spouse to tell the truth?
   Always   Mostly   Sometimes   Rarely   Never

7. Do you know where you stand on financial matters?
   Always   Mostly   Sometimes   Rarely   Never

8. Can you tell your partner what pleases you sexually?
   Always   Mostly   Sometimes   Rarely   Never

9. Are you comfortable with the way your spouse parents?

   Always   Mostly   Sometimes   Rarely   Never

10. Are you comfortable with your partner's relationship to his or her parents?

    Always   Mostly   Sometimes   Rarely   Never

11. Can you talk about death? Your partner's? Your own?

    Always   Mostly   Sometimes   Rarely   Never

Questions to Help You Begin Open Discussion

1. The thing I like most about our relationship is _____

2. The thing I value most about you is _____

3. I am proud of you when _____

4. I am bothered by you when _____

5. I believe or don't believe in _____

6. I am afraid of _____

7. I hope that _____

8. I like it when _____

9. It upsets me when _____

10. Remember the time we _____

11. I am sorry about _____

12. Your gift to me has been _____

13. Your challenge to me has been _____

14. I feel safest with you when _____

15. I feel shakiest with you when _____

16. You are most helpful when _____

17. I am sensitive about _____

18. You stop being open with me when I _____

19. I don't like to talk about _____

20. I admire that _____

21. I think we could be closer if _____

22. Last night I dreamt _____

23. I always wanted to _____

24. I think it would be fun to _____

25. I wish that we could _____

26. The ways I want you to touch me are _____

27. The ways I don't want you to touch me are _____

28. Did I ever tell you how much I like your _____

29. I am concerned that this illness interferes with _____

30. I feel closest to you when _____

31. The hardest feeling I have to deal with is _____

32. The hardest thought for me is _____

33. I want you to remember that _____

34. I believe in _____

35. I feel lucky because _____

36. I feel unlucky because _____

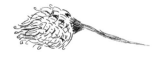

9

Showers and Love Touches: Sexuality and Other Appetites

Music heard so deeply
That it is not heard at all, but you are the music while the music lasts.

T.S. Eliot

I remember in the early days of our relationship all was passion and tousled sheets. We couldn't get enough of each other. Our bodies were warm and supple and we were irrational, insatiable, and very much in love.

Through the years, sex remained extremely important to us both. It satisfied the hunger we each had for touch, as well as for play and closeness.

Sexual Attitudes

Sexual attitudes and practices vary. One couple has intercourse daily. Another couple is satisfied with once-a-month contact. One couple experiences times of disinterest. Both are normal! Whatever you as a couple decide, whatever makes you happy, is normality for you.

One couple only assumes the missionary position. They shun oral sex. Another couple has attempted everything in the Kama Sutra. There are no absolutes. There are also no age restrictions.

Healthy sexuality is a cycle of desire, excitement, orgasm, and resolution. The phases may be interrupted at any point. You don't have to have an orgasm every time. The resolution phase will occur a bit more slowly, but this is not a disaster. Men need recovery time after orgasm. As they age, the time between erections lengthens.

Prostate cancer forced us to make treatment decisions that we knew would alter our sexual interactions. We discussed all the treatment alternatives together, knowing that ultimately the choice of treatment would be, had to be, Bob's. It was his life; it was his decision to make.

I hoped he would choose surgery. I wanted that cancer out. I viewed it as an intruder, a trespasser. Of course I wanted him the way he used to be, but I didn't care at that moment about erections, ejaculations, or orgasms. I wanted him alive.

He opted to go with radioactive seed implants rather than surgery. Bob detested the thought that the sexual part of our relationship might be over. He expressed his concern repeatedly. His prostate was enlarged, and some of our physicians tried to discourage him. He remained determined to have the seed implants. The fact was that sex, as we had known it, was over.

Choices

Helen Kaplan, M.D., Ph.D., says, "Any generally debilitating and/or painful disease will affect sexual functioning adversely. In addition endocrine disturbances which interfere with testosterone production or utilization also impair libido in both genders, and erection in the male."[22]

A radical prostatectomy surgically removes the prostate and seminal vessels. Radiation can interfere with the ability to have an erection. Chemotherapy lowers the testosterone level and that often lowers sexual desire.

Hormone therapy is not completely understood. Its effect varies. In some cases, men have desire and erections and orgasms. In other cases, they do not.

Bob asked for hormone therapy to reduce his prostate enlargement and eventually convinced his doctor that he was an appropriate candidate for seed implantation. In his case, it turned out to be a poor decision. The cancer had moved in his body with a vengeance. He required many seeds and the seeds migrated. This led to complications.

The seed radiation affected his ability to have an erection. The walls of his arteries lost their elasticity. Bob lost his sexual desire and the cancer spread. Side effects are unpredictable.

In our present health-care environment, we have to take responsibility for our medical decisions. The doctor is our advisor, but it remains essential for us to understand the ramifications of treatment. The choice is ours. What works for one person may not and often does not work for someone else.

Our love stayed strong and we would hold each other close at night, kissing away our growing fears. We experimented and tried different positions. We tried massage. We talked about our feelings.

The adversity drew us closer together in some ways. One night he said it would be all right with him if I found a lover. I told him I had a lover and his name was Bob. He was all I wanted and needed. Somewhere along the line, I turned off the switch of libido and changed my concept of what constituted sexuality. Cuddling seemed to be enough for me. Stroking seemed to be enough for him.

You Need to Know

Gathering as much information as you can on what to expect is important. Even when erection is not viable, the ability to attain the feeling of orgasm often exists. You can attain pleasure when you accept the idea of mutual stimulation and self-stimulation.

Sex helps you to feel alive. Physical caring can overcome tiredness and depression. Partners have to be willing to keep the lines of communication open. Sometimes, in the course of cancer treatment, the concept that one is no longer attractive becomes a psychological barrier. Performance anxiety will interfere with the attempt at physical closeness. You can overcome this. When a partner offers reassurance and understanding, the anxiety may subside quickly. If the anxiety persists, it may be time to seek sexual counseling. Anxiety is treatable!

By overcoming embarrassment, one can discover new ways of gratification. In our media-driven society, people often feel that the only way to reach orgasm is by having the penis inside the vagina. There are many other ways of being satisfied.

Sex therapist Helen Kaplan begins in the first session by stating, "He doesn't need to have an erection and it is not his partner's duty to make him have one. It is not a requirement to have an orgasm."

There is no such thing as failure when one realizes that pleasure may come from hands and lips and that sensual experiences don't have to be erotic.

Keeping in Touch

We experimented by stroking each other's bodies. We would focus on the belly or legs or neck. We only avoided areas that were painful and we talked to each other about what felt good and what didn't. We learned to listen to each other with our hearts.

Bob and I enjoyed each other for many months till there came a time when even gentle massage was impossible. Bob could only find relaxation and relief from his pain by taking hot baths. Then, as his disease progressed, it became increasingly difficult for him to step into or out of our deep tub.

We had enthusiastically created an elegant bathroom in our dream house, with a Jacuzzi soaking tub and a stall shower that required two steps down into an adjoining space. We had never considered the possibility that we would need handrails or easy access. We had to work out a coping routine.

He used his walker to the top step and held onto the wall while I repositioned it. He took a deep breath, then a step, then leaned on me until he could get back on his walker. A twenty-second descent took us five minutes.

As I soaped him, I would trace the body hair on his chest into swirls. I memorized the contour of his back. We were a long way from our wild days of sexual passion, but we were making love as he accepted my ministrations. It was a new kind of sexuality.

It didn't occur to me that a small bathing chore could carry so much emotion until we arrived at the time for hospice home care. When the agency offered to send a caregiver to help bathe him every other day, I snapped a refusal. I was rude.

This was my job. This was my labor of love. I was possessively clinging to this form of body contact. I didn't want a stranger to touch him. Each of us reacts in a different way. For someone else, the bath help would have seemed a relief. I saw it as an intrusion.

My sleep became fretful. I would listen to Bob's breathing throughout the night, always on the alert. I focused the same awareness I'd had as a young mother tending to my baby onto Bob. It was exhausting.

The hospice offer of help could have been a blessing, but for me it signaled another ending that I couldn't tolerate or accept. So I didn't. Bob and I resisted every phase of letting go. We mourned every change. Sometimes we cried, together and separately. Sometimes we swallowed our tears so as not to alarm each other.

It was wonderful when we were able to talk, but solitude often trapped us. Together and totally separate, locked in death's inevitability, we resisted letting go over and over again.

Other Appetites

I kept encouraging Bob to eat. I could see him getting thinner. I tried special corned beef sandwiches, ice cream, and finally Ensure. We talked to the nutritionist. She was helpful, but Bob ate less and less.

It finally occurred to me that I was part of the problem.

Food has always been a part of connecting. We socialize over meals. We show our love by preparing biscuits. Betty Crocker tells us so.

The less Bob cared about eating, the more helpless I felt. Another hard lesson. Accept that a body is wise; it knows what it needs. Badgering a patient creates one more burden. If you present meals attractively, if you check to see what seems appealing, you've done your job. Loss of appetite is not a rejection of you!

One day Bob wanted onion soup. I didn't have time to make it, but he hadn't expressed interest in any food for a long time. I called La Gare, the little French restaurant in town. Madame Gladys Praplan, the proprietor, said they were closed. My heart sank.

"Please," I said, "my husband is so ill and I think he would eat your onion soup. You make it so well."

My voice wrapped around a stifled sob. Without a pause, she said, "You come right down. I will open the restaurant." She filled my crock-pot with soup and refused to charge me for it.

Along your journey, you will find treasured moments and people full of compassion. Watch for them and savor them. This was one of mine.

Here are some practical tips to meet the challenges of frailty.

Making It Easier

Check with an occupational therapist. He or she can help you decide on which aids will make life easier. A therapist can help you find the most inexpensive ways to solve physical difficulties.

Some equipment can be borrowed. Check with hospice, the Visiting Nurse Association, home health care agencies, American Cancer Society, the Red Cross, and/or the Muscular Dystrophy Association.

If you wish to buy your equipment, check medical supply catalogs or surgical supply stores. Always check with your doctor or the hospital discharge planner before you invest. They can advise you as to what you need.

Remember that some of the durable equipment is eighty percent covered by Medicare or private insurance when it is pre-authorized by your physician. If you have state retirement or are enrolled in a union program, you may also have coverage.

Here are a few suggestions in the meantime.

1. Put a rubber mat on the shower floor.
2. Make sure your bathroom door will not lock.
3. If you have steps, edge them with nonskid tape.
4. Install grab rails if possible.
5. Lower the thermostat on your hot water faucet.
6. Get a transfer bench so that it is easier to get in and out of the tub.
7. Obtain a portable toilet seat with handrails.
8. Attach a handheld shower hose to your tub or shower faucet.
9. Install a bath bench, a real aid in either a tub or stall shower.
10. Add a pressure mattress or egg carton foam rubber to help ease bedsores.
11. Consider an easy chair with a lift in the seat.

12. Make sure that you are ready in the event of a power failure with blankets, a battery radio, candles, matches, a manual can opener, and some bottles of sterile water.

13. Make a list of general supplies and post it where you can see it so that you can easily remember to replace items you've run out of.

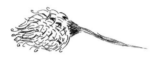

10

The Empty Chair:
Addressing Anxiety and Depression

I wake in shadow.
Neck is strained, shoulders cramped, stomach tight.
Sighs within breath stifle each move.
It will be better.
I will be better.
Hope turns darkness into dawn.
I heard that somewhere in a song but lost the words.
Forehead knotting
Hope isn't there.
Just fear and pain, twin gnomes
Huddled in my brain
Throw a switch wish to ponder something else.
Gray fog hovering, licking at the window.
Believe. Faith isn't here today.
Nobody's home.

My cat is missing. Been out all night.
Frightened, I hear baying of coyotes.
Where are you, cat?
Battle scarred cat,
Survivor, scrapper, napper
You make the best of time.
Unlike me, you live undaunted,
Uncollared, unchained.
Come home, cat. I need you here.
For I exist within translucent threads.
Of spider web: a trapped insect, a mosquito, a fly, a bee.
Naked, marinated, caught in silk thread,
Waiting to be the spider's feast.
So come home, cat. Rescue me.
I hear the sounds of bat wings.

Maryann Schacht

Bob felt too ill to attend the symphony one night. I decided to go alone. The music was beautiful but I couldn't forget the empty chair beside me. I couldn't tell you what they played that night. We had relinquished our excellent seats in the dress circle for orchestra seats on the side of the auditorium. A knot of resentment settled in my chest. I tried telling myself to stop being ridiculous. I started a pep talk about music as a direct connection between the orchestra and the listener (me). That didn't help either. That night still stands out in my memory. My aloneness crashed in my brain. "Oh Lord, please," I prayed, "let him get better!"

Depression can be a short-term or a long-term problem. It can creep up on you or suddenly strike you down. Depression is painful and can be immobilizing, no matter what form it takes. It can evolve from an appropriate grief reaction into an inappropriate, paralyzing morass. We must always address depression.

It is appropriate to mourn when you suffer a loss, whether big or small. If you lose the tiniest tip of your finger, everything changes. You no longer have the same agility in picking up tools. You may see yourself as less than perfect in appearance. The loss feels strange and takes getting used to. You act appropriately when you mourn loss. It takes time to develop a new sense of the way you are now. You may overestimate or underestimate exactly what a change means. You may forget that your amputated finger is not your essence.

Depression settles in when you inflate the importance of the body and lose touch with your soul process. You may try to distract yourself by doing busy work, or you may take the other route and give yourself the time to explore your mood from the inside. While the busy work is helpful in the short term, deeper exploration enables you to discover new facets of yourself. You know what is right for you at the moment. Trust your intuition.

More often than not, the depression is based on worrying about things that may never happen at all. No room remains for joy when catastrophic thoughts take up too much of our energy. Too often we pass through the hours of our existence ruminating about what could or should have been or, alternatively, projecting ourselves into the "awfulness" of the future. Depression can be seen in one form as generalized anxiety or in its extreme as a full-blown terror and/or all-pervasive despair.

You are suffering from depression when you lose interest in your family, your friends, and the events of the day. It is depression when you find yourself waiting for the next shoe to drop, when you are exhausted, drained, and have no hope. When you stop believing in yourself, you're depressed.

Both the past and the future are illusionary. Time spent worrying about either interferes with enjoying whatever you have on your plate at the moment. If you are eating lentil soup and your chattering mind keeps warning you that lentil soup is going to give you gastric indigestion, you certainly can't relish a mouthful. Worry never helps. Action does. You can take Beano, eat and enjoy, or stop eating the lentil soup. Taking action avoids the gas, but the ruminating did not and will not change a thing.

Depression, like illness, is an unwelcome visitor who changes all the interactive and internal dynamics of the family. For one person, it heightens fear of separation, of disappearance, of disapproval. For another, it becomes anger turned inward upon itself. Depression hangs vulnerability out on the line for all to witness. It thrives on the waves of unknown impending change. It is embarrassing. Worst of all, depression is contagious. So let's take a moment to break it down.

One component of depression is anxiety that actually does serve a purpose. It is an alarm system saying, "Be on guard. There is something amiss. There is a stranger in the house." The anxiety takes different forms, manifesting itself as either vague or particular. It can appear as a slight discomfort or as a sense of suffocation, a beating in the brain, a fever, a loud pounding heartbeat. Even in the best of cases, it is unpleasant.

When I wrote the poem calling for my cat, I was able to define the physical aspects of my depression. I experienced all of my feelings. I could break the sense of hopelessness down into pieces small enough to handle. I could do something about each of the pieces by addressing each one directly. Then, I could get a massage or take a hot bath to alleviate the pain in my neck and cramp in my shoulders. I could consider the symbolism of the cat and seek to emulate what I admired about him. I could identify my need to "clear away the fog." After writing, I felt less overwhelmed. Writing my feelings down on paper translated discomfort into something else altogether. Seeing the actual descriptive words on paper concretized my feelings and eliminated the possibility of disowning them. I experienced what I felt in the moment.

The first step is to recognize and accept that there are times when anxiety will arise. It only turns into depression when you can't see a way out. If you lose faith in your defense system, you give up any hope of mastery.

Anxiety is transient. Everything in life changes all the time. Moods come and go. Realities come and go. When you are in a low period and you want to shift your mood, allow yourself to experience whatever you are feeling fully without self-judgment. Self-criticism will only defeat your purpose. Try to express yourself in a creative activity. Drawing, painting, or composing music can change the way you feel. The art form needs to be for you alone, although many times it becomes a piece of yourself that you want to share with an audience.

You may explore all aspects of your feelings by using metaphors. You can write them, draw them, dance them, or sing them. Try drawing whatever you are feeling right now as a shape. Color it.

Try putting your feelings into movement, with or without music. Try it both ways. Find which approach works best for you.

Whenever you take an action, the act itself shows you that you are not immobilized. The feeling, bad as it may be, does not have to devastate you. You always have an option. You can always reframe the experience of your feeling. The process of describing what you are experiencing will help to pull you out of the quicksand of depression. In movement you gain a foothold on a new reality. You restart the coping process.

You have a choice about how to behave in any circumstance.

You can cry or be stoic. You can have a temper tantrum or reason gently and firmly. You can fight or accept. You have a choice.

You always have the option of repeating a behavior that is familiar. It may have worked for you in the past and you may find it useful in the present. However, if what you are doing is not working, take a risk and try something else.

If Mom didn't laugh at your jokes, it does not mean that you have no sense of humor. Just because you were told it is not OK to get angry, it does not mean that you should squash your indignation into oblivion.

An old Buddhist tale describes a monk who became concerned because his once thriving congregation was shrinking. He asked why. A disciple told him that the people no longer came because they feared a big snake that hissed at them whenever they walked up the mountain path. The monk stood up and strode down the mountain.

When he found the snake he looked directly at him and said sternly, "Your behavior is unacceptable. Stop it at once!" The snake obeyed. Soon the congregation was full and the monk was very pleased.

As the monk walked down the mountain one day, he came across the snake, totally bruised and beaten; the snake was about to breathe his last breath. "What has happened to you?" asked the monk, full of compassion.

"You told me not to hiss and I listened to you. Now the children pick up sticks and beat me, the old people throw stones at me, and I am dying," the snake answered.

The monk replied, "I told you not to hiss and strike out. I never told you not to defend yourself. Protecting yourself is not the same as bullying."

Ignoring our shadows (and we all have shadows) only lends them strength. The indigenous people of Australia gather their children around a campfire and talk to them of the Dreamtime. They say that, when you meet a monster in the Dreamtime, you must not run away. If you do, the monster will grow bigger and bigger and become more and more threatening. When you stand your ground and look him directly in the eye, the monster will shrink until you are far more powerful than he is.

Shadows and monsters hate to be ignored. The more you avoid them, the louder they shout. When you acknowledge and befriend them, you can use all the energy that they were draining from you.

Once, in a psychodrama group, a client presented the fact that a student in her class was sapping all of her strength. She described the situation in a tired, listless voice. She truly had no energy left to deal with her troublesome student. I asked her to become the student and show us all just what she was up against. Immediately she took on the strong bold stance of the defiant student and, with an impish gleam in her eye, she proceeded to bait the actor playing the part of the teacher. The energy charged through her. She really let the teacher have it. When she finally simmered down and reversed back into her teacher role, she chuckled. The change was remarkable. She had found her own energy by giving vent to her inner child "fresh kid."

Jung said that acknowledging and accepting our shadows is part of the maturation process. We open to the possibility of becoming whole each time we accept who we are.

Rose, one of my clients, came to our support group because her husband suffered from multiple sclerosis, a degenerative disease that can have periods of remission or may run a steady, progressive, downhill course.

He had been through a great deal but he was holding his own. He'd been tested and prodded with thin needles, tapped and assessed. He kept figuring the worst was still to come and sat for hours staring into space and drinking more alcohol than he should.

Rose found her world shrinking drastically. Every day she got up, made breakfast, fixed the bed, and urged Fred to do something, anything. He just lumbered over to his big leather chair and sat.

She had taken to fussing over him throughout the day. Did he want water? Was he too cold or too warm? They lived in their own apartment and both could still drive, although he refused to consider that or any other possibility. She felt lonely and bored. He didn't seem to want her company. He didn't want anyone's company.

Still it was hard for her to leave him alone in the house. So, neither of them left the apartment except to go to physician appointments or food shopping. It was a big deal for this committed housewife to consider attending a support group.

Rose believed that marriage meant absolute togetherness; the idea of taking a break felt disloyal to her. It took enormous effort to give herself the gift of two hours in a support group. It was only because the doctor had told her she would be no use at all if she didn't get a grip on her own depression that she had agreed to come.

The first time she came, she spoke very little. When she did speak, her voice was low and her words muffled. Tears at any and every statement glistened in the corners of her eyes.

"I don't think the doctors know anything. They say there is a good chance of remission, but we both know that the end is near. I'm afraid the end is near. He doesn't want strangers in the house. I don't know if I will be able to help him. I don't know where to get a wheelchair. I don't think I'll be able to get him in and out of one."

On and on she went, interpreting everything in a negative way, unwilling to consider the possibility of her husband going into a remission because she didn't want to feel disappointed if it didn't happen.

Every ache meant that the disease was getting worse. Every cramp she got in her seventy-four-year-old legs meant that she would precede him into the nursing home. On sunny days, it was too hot to go out. On rainy days, it was too dangerous. Rainy days also induced aches and pains. She felt trapped and thought being trapped was inevitable. She emanated the sighs of her partner's despair. Like a bad cold, she had caught his depression.

She needed to be jolted out of her pattern. The group members rose to the task. "You are wasting whatever time you have," said one member of the group and suggested she keep a log and write down every favorable thing she could think of between now and the next meeting.

They challenged her to notice what she cooked and how that tasted. She was told to listen for birdsong and check when and if anything surprised her on her assigned daily walk to the mailbox. They suggested she make contact with an old friend. Most important of all, she was to arrange to have someone come to visit her husband while she went out to lunch with a neighbor. She was to do that at least one time before the group met again.

With permission granted, Rose was able to make a shift in her attitude. The group acknowledged Rose's right to be separate from Fred. They let her know that she didn't have to suffer every ache and pain along with him.

She did not have to take on all of his difficulty. He had his own life to live, and he was the only one who could do that. If she continued to try to live it for him, she would add to his burden as well as her own. He needed to deal with whatever came up without projecting it onto her. She needed to develop the faith that he was a capable person and was entitled to deal with his illness in his way. Having time to replenish her resources allowed her to be more rather than less available to Fred.

Healthy spouses have to create separate time. They experience wear and tear right along with their ill partner. When the ailing person has to stay at home and the partner stays at home unwillingly, the ailing person knows it. When the healthy spouse is conflicted about going out, the replenishment is spoiled.

Both partners need to be open enough to let their partners know when they feel deprived. It is OK to say that you miss going out to a party or attending a ball game, that you are tired of "showing up" and need some alone time. This honesty enhances an honest relationship.

The patient needs separate time also. He or she needs time to assess and to grieve. He or she will benefit from facing and dealing with his or her feelings. Constant attention can be a distraction and a constant drain.

There are times when the patient will have feelings of abandonment and need to be reassured. Identifying what one wants can bring about resolution. He or she may be keeping a stiff upper lip in order to make everyone around him feel better. That can be an added burden. We may focus attention outward when the proper inclination is to withdraw and focus inward. There are decisions to be made in every waking moment. We need to explore and discuss them.

Exercise

Identify what you are feeling right this moment.

1. Ask where that feeling comes from.

2. Ask yourself what the worst part of that feeling is.

3. Decide what you can do about that.

4. Do it right now!

The more that you can define and share, the more understanding you will gain and the deeper your relationship will become.

Develop the practice of listening.

Restate what has been said in an open-ended way:

1. Are you feeling...

2. Do you mean...

3. It seems to me that...

4. Am I right about that?

It is a tenuous line to walk, but, the more open you can be, the more your partner can accept his or her upset world.

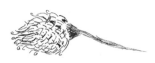

11

Money Talk: Take It out of the Shadow

The trouble with most people is that they think with their
hopes and fears or wishes rather than with their minds.

Will Durant

"I need to know exactly how much money we have and where everything is," I said, as sweetly as I could.

"Next week," he answered and looked away. "I'm pulling everything together for the accountant then."

This small exchange was fraught with all of our anxiety. His and mine.

Thoughts of a future without him had battered their way into my consciousness ever since his cancer diagnosis

I knew only too well that I allowed Bob to carry the financial end of our partnership throughout our marriage. I took the position that everything was fine as long as I had money in the bank to pay bills. Yet all along I'd recognized that I had been behaving like a child, a pre-liberated woman. Well, he enjoyed finance and I didn't, I rationalized.

Faced with an uncertain future, I felt edgy and unsure, not only of myself but of him.

Whenever I raised the subject, Bob skittered away. Tomorrow always appeared to be tomorrow. I knew he was upset. Each time I mentioned our assets, his awareness of his own mortality popped up in his mind.

Was it fair of me to hound him? How could I let him know that I thought there would come a time when I would be on my own? I'd have to know everything then, and I'd have to manage everything without him then. I didn't want to have to look for an advisor, so I stayed in his face. I could feel him bristle.

As long as I leaned on him, he could delude himself into thinking that nothing had changed. Nothing would happen to him. Nothing could happen to him. He had the erroneous belief that, since he was too important and too responsible, he must be indestructible. If I learned too much and didn't need him anymore, he would become irrelevant. This was crazy and emotional thinking. We both knew better.

We didn't discuss it out loud. I'm not altogether sure if my hypothesis was real. We were both so emotionally caught that we ignored the things that had to be said and addressed. Since both of us wanted him to continue being productive and proud, ignoring these topics was easy.

But I was scared. I knew that I absolutely had to learn the ins and outs of our affairs, and that it would be much easier now than later. I have known too many widows and widowers who had to straighten out their business affairs in the midst of grief. They had to take over financially when they could least think clearly. I didn't want that to happen to me. Finally I couldn't ignore the situation anymore.

I took a deep breath and remembered transactional analysis theory. I would no longer stay in my "child" state. I could no longer hide in my nurturing "parent" state. I needed to summon up my adult and get this difficult process under way.

The founder of transactional analysis, Eric Berne, M.D., said, "Parent, adult and child are not concepts like Superego, Ego, and Id, but phenomenological realities."[23]

Our parent state is either controlling or nurturing. It may be critical, superstitious, or cautious. The parent is the amalgamation of all the things our parents taught us and may be protective and inconsistent. At the time we learned our particular parent state, we did not censor anything. Therefore our parent state is full of admonitions and injunctions.

We accepted whatever our parents presented as life's truth. Whatever Mom and Dad said and did influenced and formed part of our parent state. If they nurtured or they criticized, we reproduce their example and their concerns. The parent state lacks spontaneity, but it comforts and heals sometimes. If your significant other feels sick and you reach out and massage his or her forehead in a loving way, that parenting action becomes a soothing balm. In many cases, parent-to-child messages build closeness. Six ego states operate in every conversation between two people. In complementary transactions, my parent addresses your parent, child, or adult or my child plays with your child, seeks guidance from your adult or enjoys "stroking" from your parent.

In the child state, we can become the pawn of our emotions. We re-experience feelings of what we encountered when very small—the fear, the anger, the vulnerability, and the intense joy. The child state can be exciting and wonderful. Sometimes it's exactly where we need to be—running on a beach, flying a kite, experiencing the gentle wind on our faces. When our playful child transacts with our partner's happy adventurous child, the results are joyful.

The adult state evolves from our own original thought and experience. This is the evaluator, that part of us that weighs and measures and then makes up our own minds. The adult state mediates between the injunctions of the parent and the reactivity of the child.

We must develop a strong adult in order to have a satisfying life. Yet the adult state isn't always the best way to be. Weighing and measuring everything sometimes seems a drag, inappropriate in the midst of sexual passion and interfering with a full appreciation of experiencing the here and now.

All three states make up who we are and how we respond to others in every transaction and interaction. All of us ought to be able to move back and forth between our parent, adult, and child parts at will. When we don't use all the states, we become rigid. We need to relate to each other from different positions.

In this particular situation, my adult would have to talk directly to his adult in order for us to reach any resolution. If I approached Bob about our financial affairs from my child position, he would probably respond from his parent position. I would experience whatever he said as a put-down, in either a docile or rebellious, foot-stamping response. It just wouldn't work if I started from the wrong position. Neither of us could end up feeling satisfied.

If I was accusatory of his handling of our affairs, he was likely to respond from his child state. That meant anger in any of its many manifestations: yelling, withdrawal, sarcasm, avoidance. It was a no-win situation and I would not end up with the vital information I needed. It would require my adult to meet his adult for our finances to be discussed in a meaning ful manner.

I began by sitting myself down and formulating a list of questions. I was painfully aware of how little I knew. My task required both discipline and thought.

Where did we keep our important papers—in the safe deposit box, in the upstairs desk drawer, where? I was pretty sure that the mortgage papers and our marriage license were in the vault, but I didn't know about the insurance policies. I didn't even know if our coverage was adequate. I didn't know what the coverage was.

After I finished beating myself up, I decided to get organized. I began by listing everything that made up our net worth, our assets and our liabilities. What did we owe? What were we owed? What would I have to know and need to do if Bob were to die? I gasped at the thought and got on with the job.

I discovered that it was necessary to have fifteen to twenty copies of the death certificate so that all the insurance companies could be notified. I wanted documentation from Bob as to what he thought I ought to do about the house, partnerships, and gifts to the children. I wanted some sense of what our cash flow was and how to manage raising funds if I needed them.

It took a while, but I organized lists of the information I'd need. Use the following materials to help you through this difficult process.

Getting Organized

Bank Accounts		Branch		Account Number

Savings Accounts		Branch		Account Number

Checking Accounts		Branch		Account Number

Loans		Where		Account Number

Stocks	Shares		Owner	Orig. Cost		Value	Total

Bonds	Type	Owner	Interest Rate	Due Date

Government Securities

List of Tax Related Accounts	
Pension Plan	
IRA or Keough Plan	
Taxes	
Past Tax Returns	
Canceled Checks	

Real Estate	Description	Approximate Value
Title Policy		
Mortgage Documents		
Tax Assessments		
Trust Deeds		
Real Estate Notes		
Rental Agreements		
Rental Receipts		
Receipts for Repairs		
Receipts for Improvements		

Insurance Type	Policy Number	Expiration Date
Life Insurance		
Homeowner's		
Auto		
Major Medical		
Life		
Disability		
Basic Medical Care		
Basic Hospital Expense		
Basic Surgical Services		
Medicare Supplement		
Vehicles		
Registration		
Proof of Ownership		
Loan Agreement		
Loan Payment Records		
Lease Agreement		
Repair Records		
Cash Flow		

Credit Card Issuer	Account Number	Expiration Date	Telephone Number to Report Loss

Safe Deposit Box	Location	Key Location	Persons Authorized to Enter

Power of Attorney	
Name	
Address	
Phone	
Cell Phone	
email	

List of Annuity Contacts	
Social Security	
Civil Service	

Important Papers	
Birth Certificate	
Marriage Certificate	
Divorce Papers	
Military Papers	
Social Security Card	
Children's Birth Certificates (if they are under age)	
Wills	
Trusts	

24

With the lists in front of us, the long-dreaded conversation took place without a hitch. We then put together the following list of important advisors that either of us might need to call at some future date.

Attorney   **Firm**
Address
Phone

Accountant   **Firm**
Address
Phone

Banker   **Bank**
Address
Phone

Life Insurance Agent   **Firm**
Address
Phone

Auto Insurance Agent   **Firm**
Address
Phone

Homeowner's Insurance Agent   **Firm**
Address
Phone

Investment Advisor   **Firm**
Address
Phone

Finding the right advisors takes a little effort but is worth the time spent. You will need to interview each of them in the same way you did when finding your physician.

Check on whether you are comfortable talking to the prospective advisor. Don't be trapped into a relationship because you want to be nice. Make sure you understand what the charges will be.

Ask about their specialty, their education, and how long they have worked in their field. Ask whom will you will actually deal with. If you will be dealing with an associate, state that you want to interview him or her. Make sure that you feel comfortable with him or her.

Remember that you are the customer and you have the right and the obligation to stay in charge.

You always have the right of decision. Your financial health is important. Being a knowledgeable consumer is the best way to keep your financial affairs in good shape.

Irving Rothenberg, CPA, a well-respected financial planner in Santa Rosa, California, suggests developing a notebook with all financial data, cash flow, business issues, estate taxes, and considerations for alternate planning in it.

You should also include a letter to your spouse or other survivors.

Sample Letter

Date

To my survivors:

I have put a great deal of thought into planning for your future and I want to share my priorities with you at this time.

First and foremost I want to make sure that Olivia is financially secure. Second I want to maintain harmony with the family, protect and maintain the mail order business, and save on our taxes.

I have set up a trust for Olivia so that she can continue to live in our house if she chooses to do so and will not have to alter her lifestyle in any way.

My intent has been to be fair and equitable to you all. This is almost impossible, however, since we have several assets, which have strong emotional ties and/or are hard to value.

At my death the stock of Haverstraw, Inc. will be sold to my partner Alfred as per our Buy/Sell Agreement. The payout will be over a two-year period. I suggest that you invest the money in stable mutual funds.

Our assets are difficult to value and in order to save as much on taxes as possible we have assessed them at the lowest possible yet reasonable figure.

If you have any questions, please consult my accountant.

Our Estimated Tax Liability

The Federal and State estate and death taxes as of _____ on the death of _____ would be approximately:

Federal tax due	$ _____
State tax due	$ _____

This tax was based on numerous assumptions and estimates as of the date indicated above. The actual fair market value of assets on the date of death will most likely change the amount of tax due. The actual amount of tax will also be affected by changes in the tax law since the date of this computation. Other factors, such as asset acquisitions, gifts given or received, or changes in the beneficiaries, could affect the amount of tax due.

| Average Monthly Cash Flow Worksheet ||
Category	Amount
Income	
Dividends	
Employment	
Interest	
Pension	
Real Estate	
Social Security	
Outlay	
Clothing	
Contributions	
Debts	
Education	
Entertainment	
Food	
Housing	
Income Tax	
Insurance	
Medical	
Miscellaneous	
Pension Distribution	
Property Tax	
Transportation	
Utilities	
Other	

Irregular Expenditure Worksheet		
Item	Amount	Month Due
Charitable Contributions		
Club Membership		
Estimated Tax		
Exercise of Stock Options		
Furniture		
Holiday Gifts		
Home Improvements		
Maintenance		
Homeowner's/Renter's Insurance		
Life Insurance		
Notes		
Other Insurance		
Property Taxes		
Retirement Plan Contributions		
Seasonal Fuel/Electricity		
Tuition		
Vacation		
Other		
Other		

Money issues are core issues. They tap into the envious part of us. They tap into insecurity and outright fear. You both may have a strong reaction after completing this chapter assignment. That is to be expected.

Very few of us can take a hard look at our finances and our lifestyles in a detached manner. You might find old resentments rising to the surface. You may focus on what you would have liked to have acquired or completed, but if you allow yourself to shine a light directly into this particular shadow, you will find that you become closer and more supportive of one another than ever before. Stay open and loving and persistent.

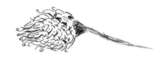

12

Hard Decisions: Medical Power of Attorney

Courage the footstool of virtues,
upon which they stand.

Robert Louis Stevenson

Bob believed that if and when he could no longer participate in an active life, he would choose to die. He was clear about that. Being on dialysis, he had the option. He could just choose not to go for treatment. But, as he began to fail, he kept pushing back the boundaries of his timeline. At first he said it would be when he could no longer drive. Next it was when he could no longer play bridge, and then when he could no longer attend the men's group. The men moved their meeting to our house and the dialysis refusal vanished. He who said he would never tolerate tubes learned to live with a colostomy.

It was his decision to make. Finally I sat down with him and asked what his outside limit was. I would help him do whatever he wanted to do, but he needed to put it in writing. Finally, he said he would tell me when he could no longer tolerate what he had to face. If he became brain-dead and couldn't express his wishes, he wanted me to take him off of anything that kept him alive mechanically.

"The children need to see that in writing," I said. I reminded him of the terrible situation I'd had with one of my client families.

When Renee first became ill, she told her husband Joseph that she didn't want to be kept alive artificially. Saying that she didn't want any heroic measures was as far as she went. No one thought it necessary to put anything in writing. Renee knew that Joseph needed to talk things over before she made her decision. Throughout their married life, she had been the one who said, "Let's do it."

She had the closest tie with her son Richard and wanted to give him power of attorney, but worried about how Joseph would feel if she designated power of attorney to their son. So she did nothing.

When Renee's cancer weakened her to the point that she could no longer swallow, she was placed on intravenous feeding. Then she stopped breathing and a respiratory machine was brought in. Renee's tough constitution kept functioning while her brain stopped. The doctors were in charge.

The family felt bewildered. They all loved her deeply, but each loved her in their own ways. Ways differed. Richard felt his mother should be allowed to die. His father and his sister Barbara clung to the possibility of recovery and wanted everything that could be done. They wanted her life preserved at all cost.

The medical staff agreed. The doctor in charge clearly stated that he was in the business of saving lives. He would want to fibrillate Renee's heart and restart her breathing, even though she had no hope of recovery.

Joseph, Renee's husband, stayed frozen. He paced the floor outside her hospital room but rarely went in to see her. He felt Renee was suffering unnecessarily, but the thought of a world without Renee overwhelmed him.

He listened to his children squabble and watched and agonized and did nothing. Renee had always been so capable. He needed her to make the decision. He found himself wishing she would just let go and let them get on with their lives. He hated himself for his wishes.

Could this family's dilemma have been eased if Renee had addressed her goals and priorities ahead of time? Of course!

If Renee had sat down with Joseph, Richard, and Barbara to spell out her desires and assign durable power of attorney to someone she trusted to carry out her wishes, they would all have felt freer to abide by her choices. Nothing is ever simple, but decisions are much less complicated when the whole family knows exactly what the patient wants.

In our situation, Bob gave me power of attorney over his health care. He did not want to be kept alive when he could no longer think. That was his bottom line. No two people will have the same bottom line. The important thing is to find out what you both think and explore those issues that have a bearing on your answers

The following section is designed to help the person you are caring for clarify his or her values.[25]

Clarifying Your Values

Let us begin with the way that you are both relating to your health care team.

1. Do you like your doctor?
2. Do you trust his or her opinions?
3. Do you want to leave the treatment decisions to him or her?

4. How do you feel about your:
   → nurse?
   → therapist?
   → social worker?
   → minister, priest or rabbi?
5. Is there something you want to address with any of them?
6. If so, what interferes with your doing so?

Independence/Dependence

1. Do you pride yourself in doing things for yourself?
2. Have you learned how to ask for help?
3. Are you able to take in and accept other people's desire to help? If not, what previous patterning makes it hard for you to do that?
4. If your ability to do for yourself lessens, in what way will it affect your self-image?
5. How do you feel about life if dependency becomes a part of it?

Your Support System

1. Do you believe that your family and/or friends are or will be supportive of your present or future medical decisions?
2. Have you made any arrangements for a family member or friend to make medical decisions for you now or in the future? If so, under what circumstances?
3. Are you comfortable with whom you have chosen?
4. Do you have any business, legal, or personal matters that feel unfinished at this time? What do you need to do in order to put your affairs in order?
5. What do you believe about the way you would handle illness, dying, death?

Religion

1. What is your religious background?
2. How does it affect your view of illness, dying, and death?
3. Do you find comfort in your religious or nonreligious beliefs?
4. Do you pray? Are there special ceremonies or liturgies that you find helpful?
5. What else can you find that might be helpful and meaningful?
6. Have you read about, practiced, or are you open to the concept of mind-body medicine?

Home and Hearth

1. Is your current environment comfortable?
2. Do you need to make physical changes in it? How can you arrange to do that?
3. Are you considering moving or having someone come to live with you? What are the pros and cons?

Finances

1. Is money for your care a problem?
2. Do you hesitate to spend money on yourself?
3. Are you concerned about the financial impact your care is having on your family? Have you discussed your concerns?

Treatment Considerations

If a treatment is painful or invasive but offers a reasonable hope for a good outcome, would you agree to it? If the chances are slim and the results are going to be problematic, do you want to consider it anyway? In coming to a conclusion you might want to consider the impact the treatment will have on your

→ relief from pain
→ ability to experience relationships
→ ability to engage in favorite activities
→ ability to think
→ ability to communicate
→ financial costs
→ suffering and anxiety to others
→ reconciliation and tying up loose ends
→ control of bodily functions
→ ability to move about
→ privacy
→ religious needs

I realize it is difficult even to face the possibility of dying. The following statements have been helpful to other people. Adapt or adopt them as you see fit. Add to them. Subtract from them. Feel free to explore. I suggest that you keep a pad and pencil handy and make notes as you go along. Keep on communicating.

→ In case of doubt, I want you to extend my life.
→ I want only those treatments that offer reasonable hope of restoring me to a condition that my loved ones think would be acceptable to me.
→ I do, or do not, want treatment if there is only a remote chance it might help me.
→ I want treatment decisions made with consideration of my overall condition and the treatment's ability to improve this.

- ✦ I want sufficient pain medication to keep me free of pain even if the dosage necessary might shorten my life.
- ✦ I want the cost of treatment and the financial impact on my family or community to be considered when making decisions.
- ✦ If I lose consciousness and have no reasonable hope of regaining it, I want all treatment stopped (including food and fluids).
- ✦ I want my loved ones and professionals to make decisions about my care the way they think I would make them, if I were able.

Now that you have put thinking time into identifying how you want to manage your illness, take the next hour to put it in writing. You can use the following form if you wish. Make sure that whatever form you develop is dated and witnessed by two people who are not related to you. They should not be beneficiaries of your estate nor should your physician be a witness. Put a copy of your living will in your vault or other safe place and give a copy to your physician and/or attorney of health care.

Sample Living Will

Declaration made this _____ day of _____, 20_____
I, _____ declare and make known to my family, physician and others my instructions and wishes regarding my future health care. I direct that all health care decisions to accept or refuse treatment, service or procedure used to diagnose, treat or care for my physical or mental condition and decisions to provide, withhold or withdraw life-sustaining measures, be made in accordance with the statements in this document. This instruction shall take effect in the event I am unable to make my own health care decisions, as determined by the physician who has primary responsibility for my care and any necessary confirming determinations. I direct that this document become part of my permanent medical records.

The following are samples of statements you might want to include. Which one expresses your wish?

Statement 1

I direct that all medically appropriate measures be provided to sustain my life regardless of my physical or mental condition.

Statement 2

There are circumstances in which I would not want my life to be prolonged by further medical treatment. In these circumstances, life-sustaining measures should not be initiated and if they have been, they should be discontinued. I recognize this is likely to hasten my death. In the following, I specify the circumstances in which I would choose to forego life-sustaining measures.

If you have chosen Statement 2, please initial each of the statements (a, b, c) with which you agree:

a. I realize that there may come a time when I am diagnosed as having an incurable and irreversible illness, disease or condition. If this occurs, and my attending physician and at least one (1) additional physician who has personally examined me determine that my condition is terminal, I direct that life-sustaining measures which would only serve to prolong my dying be withheld or discontinued. I also direct that I be given all medically appropriate care necessary to make me comfortable and to relieve pain.

b. If there should come a time when I become permanently unconscious and it is determined by my attending physician and at least one (1) additional physician with appropriate expertise who has personally examined me that I have totally and irreversibly lost consciousness and my capacity for interaction with other people and my surroundings, I direct that life-sustaining measures be withheld or discontinued. I understand that I will not experience pain or discomfort in this condition, and I direct that I be given all medically appropriate care necessary to provide for my personal hygiene and dignity.

c. I realize that a time may come when I am diagnosed as having an incurable and irreversible illness, disease, or condition that may not be terminal. My condition may cause me to experience severe and progressive deterioration and/or a permanent loss of capacities and faculties I value highly. If, in the course of my medical care, the burdens of continued life with treatment become greater than the benefits I experience, I direct that life-sustaining measures be withheld or discontinued. I also direct that I be given all medically appropriate care necessary to make me comfortable and to relieve pain.

Additional Instructions

By this directive I inform those who may become entrusted with my health care of my wishes and intend to ease the burden of decision making which this responsibility may impose. I understand the purpose and effect of this document and sign it knowingly, voluntarily and after careful deliberation.

_____

Name

_____

Address

_____

City   State

Communicate

Talk over your will with your family. Make sure that everything is clearly spelled out and that you have chosen a person who will carry out your intentions to be your durable power of attorney for health care. Remember he or she can only make decisions if and when you are unable to make them for yourself. He or she will be limited by your specifications and whatever restrictions imposed by the law of your state.

Your living will as well as the durable power of attorney remains in effect indefinitely or unless you have a change of mind. You can reverse your will or replace your agent by notifying him or her, family members, your physician, or other health care providers. It is always best to do that in writing, but it can be done orally.

Your attorney will want to make decisions consistent with your desires. He or she is designated to act "in your best interest." To avoid confusion (and court proceedings), consider how and what you feel about the following statement of wants. Agree or disagree. Cross out anything that doesn't fit for you. This document should be attached to your Durable Power of Attorney for Health Care.

Addendum to Durable Power of Attorney for Health Care

1. If I am comatose and the physicians feel my condition is permanent, I wish to have:

Mechanical ventilation or respiration?	❑ Yes	❑ No
Kidney dialysis?	❑ Yes	❑ No
Cardiopulmonary resuscitation?	❑ Yes	❑ No
Radiation treatment?	❑ Yes	❑ No
Major or minor surgery?	❑ Yes	❑ No
Blood transfusions?	❑ Yes	❑ No
Antibiotics?	❑ Yes	❑ No
Chemotherapy?	❑ Yes	❑ No
Food and water?	❑ Yes	❑ No

2. If I have an incurable or terminal condition with no reasonable hope of survival I want:

Mechanical ventilation or respiration?	❑ Yes	❑ No
Kidney dialysis?	❑ Yes	❑ No
Cardiopulmonary resuscitation?	❑ Yes	❑ No
Radiation treatment?	❑ Yes	❑ No
Major or minor surgery?	❑ Yes	❑ No
Blood transfusions?	❑ Yes	❑ No
Antibiotics?	❑ Yes	❑ No
Chemotherapy?	❑ Yes	❑ No
Food and water?	❑ Yes	❑ No

3. If I have lost the capacity to maintain a life of dignity and cannot respond to my surroundings in any way, I want:

Mechanical ventilation or respiration? ❑ Yes ❑ No

Kidney dialysis? ❑ Yes ❑ No

Cardiopulmonary resuscitation? ❑ Yes ❑ No

Radiation treatment? ❑ Yes ❑ No

Major or minor surgery? ❑ Yes ❑ No

Blood transfusions? ❑ Yes ❑ No

Antibiotics? ❑ Yes ❑ No

Chemotherapy? ❑ Yes ❑ No

Food and water? ❑ Yes ❑ No

4. In order for my attorney-in-fact to decide in an appropriate manner I want her or him to take into account my ability to remember:

General information? ❑ Yes ❑ No

Life events? ❑ Yes ❑ No

Awareness of my surroundings? ❑ Yes ❑ No

Ability to recognize caregivers, friends and loved ones? ❑ Yes ❑ No

Ability to control bodily functions? ❑ Yes ❑ No

Ability to speak, to understand, to communicate in any way? ❑ Yes ❑ No

Ability to comprehend what is happening around me? ❑ Yes ❑ No

Ability to take pleasure in anything from the tree outside the window to a child's birthday party? ❑ Yes ❑ No

5. I wish to be as free of pain as possible even if that means administration of narcotics in doses high enough to dull awareness or shorten my life?   ❏ Yes   ❏ No

6. I wish caring and supportive nursing care and medical care to relieve pain and suffering including narcotics even if my respiration is depressed?   ❏ Yes   ❏ No

7. I want food and fluids offered as long as I am conscious?   ❏ Yes   ❏ No

8. If I am not conscious I want moist sponges to moisten my lips and relieve dehydration?   ❏ Yes   ❏ No

9. When I am deceased I want any of my usable organs or tissue to be donated to the organ bank?   ❏ Yes   ❏ No

10. I agree to autopsy if my physicians feel it would be helpful?   ❏ Yes   ❏ No

_____
Signature   Date

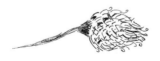

13

Hoofbeats and Prayerbeats

More things are wrought by prayer
Than this world dreams of.

Alfred Lord Tennyson

To keep my sanity, I began dressage lessons. I went twice a week and practiced for an hour with a superb horse trainer and a beautiful mare named Margarita. I'm not sure whether it was the trainer's concentration on my riding behaviors or the remarkable ability of the horse to sense my mood, but I would go home feeling as if I could face anything.

Riding became a meditation. I had no fear and neither did Margarita. A sense of safety enveloped both of us. The trust built each time we circled the ring. For the space of an hour there was total communication between that horse and me. She would respond to the simplest cue, whether it was the slightest kick to her rib or my fingers tightening on the reins.

Riding became my prayer time.

The Native American people used to say that a circle was the path to understanding life's mysteries. Energy is in every round. We see the world through eyes that are orbs. The sun and moon and the stars appear round. Birds' nests are round. Seasons follow one another, melting into each other, becoming a circle. The shaman created medicine wheels to represent an individual's universe. That riding ring was mine.

The amazing thing about meditation is that we can attain it in so many forms and places. All of us benefit when we quiet ourselves physically. It is in that calm space that prayer appears.

Help me to find the way
To love and keep faith in
This moment
This horse
This day
In my own Humanity and Frailty
Let love grow and overflow
Beyond ego and pain
Beyond error in thinking
Beyond thinking at all
Help me find the courage
To let go and trust
In life's pattern.

Maryann Schacht

As we relinquish the idea that we can control destiny we develop a relaxation response. It happens whether or not we believe in God. Try it.

From the deep bass voice of our innermost feelings we can connect with a spiritual self.

One day as I dismounted from Margarita, my friend asked me if Bob would be amenable to a healing service. She had great faith in her Episcopal minister and felt he'd worked miracles for many people.

I said I'd ask. Bob, as I have often said, was a Jewish pragmatist. I couldn't guess what his response would be. He surprised me when he said, "Sure. A service can't hurt and it might help." A week later we joined our friends at a beautiful little church in Calistoga, California. A large open-faced man in a brown cassock greeted us. He looked like an oversized Friar Tuck. He was warm and welcoming and said he would be ready to receive us in half an hour. Would we walk the labyrinth in the meantime?

Bob couldn't handle the labyrinth. "You go," he said. The labyrinth was carefully laid out in the courtyard of the church. The segments wound around from the outer entrance to the center and then with a slight turn from the center to the exit. I tried to move slowly. One easy step at a time.

Concentrating hard, I attempted to recapture the feeling of my riding circle prayer space. It didn't work. I was much too aware of Bob watching me. It all felt forced and unnatural. I couldn't find a way to empty my mind.

Lead me in thy truth; and teach me,
For thou art the God of my salvation;
For thee I wait all the day long (Psalm 25:5)

The words and admonitions kept racing until I gave up and let it be.

When the priest motioned us to come inside, he asked if we'd been baptized. Bob said no.

He responded that it didn't matter. Would Bob kneel at the step to the altar? Bob did. The priest read passages from the Old Testament with a little bit of Matthew thrown in. It was obvious that he reached across our different religions in a loving way. Then he walked over to Bob and asked if he could bless him.

Bob looked up and answered, "I'd be honored. No man is so rich that he cannot welcome a blessing." The priest placed his hands on Bob's head and then asked if Bob would bless him back. Bob did. Those two men met in spirit in that moment.

Later on Bob said, "Next time you get the idea of having a healing service, do it for yourself. You need it more than I do."

I think he was right. Bob had a way of making peace with himself. He could meditate without being a believer. I have to struggle with a constantly chattering mind. I have to pray.

So What about Prayer?

How does it work? People have been praying for centuries, but what is it that they actually do when they pray?

They allow themselves to become aware of the wonder of our world. They work to connect with the part of themselves that reflects the beauty in being alive.

Larry Dossey, M.D., a physician by training and a leading figure in the efficacy of prayer, says, "In this society prayer is often conceptualized as talking out loud or silently to a white male cosmic parent figure, in English."[26] He doesn't believe in that concept. Dossey feels (as I do) that it is far too narrow.

People around the world pray in many different ways. They sway back and forth at the Western wall, light candles in a church, fly prayer flags in Tibet, face Mecca, and dance to drum beats.

Buddhists don't have a personal God. They offer their prayers to the Universe. To each person, God is different. God is white and black, male and female, internal and external, a force of nature, nature itself. The diversity of belief is testimony that prayer can be accomplished in many places and in many ways.

Sufis dance their prayers. Africans drum and sing and shout theirs. The movement leads to meditation and quiet. Then the meditation leads back to reengagement in activity. It is a continuum.

My time riding Margarita was both active prayer and meditation.

Mystic Thomas Merton often said, "he prayed by breathing." Being aware of breath is a central part of many religions. Instinctively we human beings focus on that which sustains us. Breath does that.

"Prayer is communication with the Absolute."

Prayer is when you address God. Meditation is when you listen for the reply.

"Praying for oneself or others makes a scientifically measurable difference in recovering from illness or trauma," Dossey says.

How Does It Work?

Today's scientists keep searching to explain why opening the mind and heart in prayer appears to prolong life, repair hearts, and correlate to spontaneous remissions. They don't have an answer to how it works, but they do have anecdotal as well as statistical evidence that it does work. While no one has been able to isolate a discrete chemical substance in the bloodstream, numerous studies indicate a direct association between faith and health. Daniel J. Benor, M.D.,[27] has written four volumes on healing research, citing nearly 150 studies. Over half of the studies show that prayer does help.

Elandur Haraldson and Thorstien Thorsteinsson did one study in which they asked participants to focus their prayers to enhance the growth of yeast placed in petri dishes. Two spiritual healers, one physician who believed in spiritual healing, and four unconvinced students were asked to focus their attention on the yeast. The students were not healers and not particularly interested in prayer. Surprise! Intention accelerated the growth rate.

Harold G. Koenig, M.D., author of *The Healing Power of Faith*, believes that faith exploration is medicine's last frontier. In his book, Koenig discusses an experiment conducted by Randolf Byrd, M.D., at San Francisco General Hospital.[28] The study divided heart patients into two groups for ten months. One group received intercessory prayer from a group of ministers and laypeople. The other group had no one praying for them.

Those prayed for had fewer complications. Those prayed for did not have as many infections requiring antibiotics (3 vs. 16). Those prayed for had a lower risk of pulmonary edema (6 vs. 18). There was a significantly different need to insert a tube into the throat to prevent cardiac arrest (0 vs. 12). Those prayed for were two-and-a-half times less likely to have heart failure!

At St. Luke's Hospital in Kansas City, Missouri, William Harris, Ph.D.[29] conducted a study on 1,000 heart patients. The patients were divided on a random basis. Half of the group received prayers from five Christian volunteers. The other half received no prayers. None of the patients knew that they were the objects of the study. The group that received prayers healed eleven percent better. Researchers went on to experiment with enzymes, fungi, bacteria, mice, chickens, and a variety of cells in petri dishes.[30] The results were amazing. Cells and enzymes don't pray, as far as we know; yet they grew faster when prayer energy was directed their way.

Dr. Koenig also references Dr. Thomas Oxman's study in which 237 patients had open-heart surgery and were studied for six months postoperative.[31] Twelve percent of the cardiac patients who did not attend church regularly died; five percent who prayed regularly died. An Israeli study done in 1993 followed 10,000 civil servants for twenty-six years. They found that Orthodox Jews were less likely to die of cardiovascular problems than non-believers.[32]

In 1995 a study at Dartmouth College in Hanover, New Hampshire, monitored 250 open-heart surgery patients and concluded that people who had religious connections and social support were twelve times less likely to die than people without those ties.

At Duke University a study on depression of 1,000 patients from 1987 to 1989 revealed that those with prayer practices coped better than those without. The form of the prayer doesn't seem to matter, as long as one employs an attitude of prayerfulness and empathy.

Perhaps the cited studies have brought you to a place of determination. You want to pray but you haven't got the hang of it. It feels awkward. It takes time and patience to develop a habit. How do we begin?

You have to explore what works for you. Mantras help some people. Focusing on a candle, repeating the name of Jesus or the word Shalom may help to bring you into the quiet awesome space of prayer. We all struggle with distraction. When I walked the labyrinth I was not able to reach a state of prayer. I kept getting caught up in the busyness of my mind.

Even exemplary John Donne, seventeenth-century poet and priest, said, "I throw myself down in my chamber, and I call in, and invite God, and his angels thither, and when they are there, I neglect God and his Angels, for the noise of a fly, for the rattling of a coach, for the whining of a door."

It will take at least a few weeks to settle in and develop the habit of prayer. Be patient with yourself. Some folks find it useful to go on a retreat. Some find it comforting and easier if they join a religious community. Your way may be solitary. You don't have to be religious to pray. Belief sometimes follows practice, just as practice may follow belief.

Buddhist Kalu Rinpoche says, "If a hundred people sleep and dream, each of them will experience a different world in his dream. Everyone's dream might be said to be true, but it would be meaningless to ascertain that only one person's dream was the true world and all others were fallacies. There is truth for each perceiver according to the karmic patterns condition-ing his perceptions."

Prayer and/or meditation is available to everyone, caregiver as well as care receiver. My own particular favorite prayer is from a song.

May I find the courage to make my life a blessing. Amen.

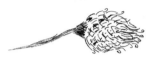

14

The Ending Time

One short sleep past, we wake eternally, and death shall be no more.

John Donne, Holy Sonnets, Number 5

Bob's face was ashen the day I helped our nurse carry him up the steps, but his determination remained strong. Once inside, he used the walker to get himself to the dining room table and tried to listen to our son Woody talk about a business deal.

I could see his mind beginning to wander and suggested he lie down. "I'm fine," he said gruffly. He struggled to concentrate, but he didn't have the energy. Finally he gave in and said that he was tired.

I asked if he wanted something to eat. He shook his head in refusal. "I'll just go sit in my chair," he said.

I could see how weak he was. My emotions froze. I knew I had to stay calm. I couldn't allow myself to see how afraid I was for him and for myself.

Bob had refused to use the hospital bed. He wanted to remain next to me in his own bed as long as possible. Our bed was built low to the floor and I struggled to help him in and out. His wish was important. I honored it as long as I could.

This time, he didn't protest as I moved him toward the hospital bed. I could feel the sea change and I told myself not to panic. Steady. Breathe. Steady.

As Bob settled into bed our Corgi, Me Too, scampered in and posted himself underneath. Our second dog, Roo, took up a position nearby and then our cat, Wellington, sat on the steps leading to the bedroom. From that time on, none of the animals would leave their posts. Me Too let out a soft yelp.

I told the family to go home. Concerned, they said they would come back if I needed them at any time, day or night. I knew they meant it. I didn't want to participate in a conversation. It seemed better for us to be on our own.

That night Bob's breathing became heavier. I called hospice for advice and they said to use the oxygen tank. Bob didn't want it, but I was able to persuade him that it would help. He motioned me to leave the room. He said he wanted to be left alone. When I protested, he said quietly, "I have to do this alone."

Because I needed to stay busy, I went to get him a glass of water. He tried to drink it to please me. He had trouble swallowing. I went back to the kitchen for a straw.

When I reentered the room I saw him kick, clench his fists, and sit up straight. He seemed to be pushing something or someone away. I went to him, put my arms around him, and told him I was there and everything was all right. He shook his head.

Then he went limp. No response. He drifted into a coma. The night passed. The next day friends came to visit, but I don't remember them being there. What I do remember are the animals. They stayed in their respective positions. Occasionally, Me Too would lick Bob's hand. Now and then Roo would whimper.

I went to put a wet cloth on Bob's head. Then I heard a rattling sound and he was gone. It was over.

After the long four-year struggle, he had left in his own way. Two-fisted and kicking. From birth to coma. He was who he was and he was one of a kind.

Me Too let out a yelp and licked his hand. Roo and Wellington didn't move. I did. I called hospice and our angel nurse Steve came as soon as he could. So did my son Woody.

Steve took charge in a reassuringly competent manner. He asked if we wanted to bathe Bob's body. I didn't think twice, but Woody hesitated for a moment. Steve encouraged him. "It will be fine," he said.

We used warm soapy water and cleaned Bob thoroughly. The last caress.

With a lump in my throat, my dark humor took over and I suggested dressing him in a tuxedo. He was an informal man, and he would always tell me that what he wore was none of my business. I was not supposed to wear him as if he were my corsage.

Keening a little, saying our last goodbyes, we dressed him in a sport shirt and loose pants. What we did there was healing and represented the beginning of acceptance.

Woody said later that it had felt so right. The act of bathing had washed his fear of death away. He had become part of the natural process of life and death. He was glad he'd been there, not only for me but also for himself.

So often we disconnect ourselves from the dying process. Our loved ones are attended by new acquaintances in a hospital setting. They often die without us present and are moved quickly to the mortuary to be embalmed and dressed by someone they never saw before. When we finally see them again, they look like plastic models of themselves. The spirit that made them who they were is no longer there.

I am grateful for the hospice way. It is so difficult to let go. Being there and using my hands helped me enormously.

I left Bob's wedding ring on his finger. Even though he had decided on cremation, I knew he would want his ring. He loved it so, with all its scratches and signs of wear. He often said the dents symbolized our long commitment to each other.

The arrival of the hearse stunned me. I felt as though someone had kicked me in my abdomen. They drove Bob away.

He was gone.

I was alone.

I was a widow.

Our house didn't feel like home any more. I made up my mind to list it for sale immediately. I couldn't, wouldn't, stay out there on the hill without Bob. Although I knew as a therapist it is better to wait before making huge decisions, I needed to move into some sort of action right then.

I went into my office, called my out-of-town family and friends, and then wrote my eulogy. Putting words down on paper always helps me gain perspective. I didn't know if I could say my words out loud, but I knew that I had to write them.

Farewell

My friend, my partner, my love, you enriched my life for over twenty-five years.

Now, I have to say farewell to you.

My man of clenched fists, always analyzing your way through this crazy, mixed-up world.

You have been my ballast, my rudder.

I will miss you.

I miss you now although I know you are and always will be a part of me forever.

On the day you left, a rainbow stretched across the sky.

I thought of it as a welcome bridge appropriate for you, always a builder of bridges.

May you take that bright-colored path and wait for me.

In time I will meet you there.

I love you.

That was all I could manage. It was enough.

We Each Have Our Own Way of Grieving

Some of us become compulsive; others become immobilized. Some of us cry. Some of us freeze. Our modus operandi is not the measure of our love. Judging others or ourselves simply makes the process more difficult.

We each have our own way of memorializing the people we love. This is why we have developed rituals. Memorial services bring us a sense of closure.

Funerals can bring families together, underscoring that individuals also belong to a group. We are not alone. Losing sight of our support systems is easy during the grief process. A congregation reassures us. A community helps us to feel connected to something larger than ourselves. Rituals put a period on one stage of life and catapult us into the inevitable new circumstances.

People all over the world have developed rituals that commit their dead to the elements: water, fire, earth, and air. Aleuts walked out onto the ice. Tibetans were dissected and offered to vultures as the people of the air. Hindus and Buddhists commit dead bodies to fire. Europeans have placed their corpses in the earth. Many people dispose of bodies and cremains in water.

Poems and psalms and song put cries into words, and then we move on. Slowly we come to grips. One part of life ends. Another begins.

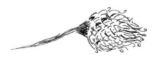

15

I Still Can't Read a Map: Going On

When Bob died, his ninety-two-year-old mother showed up at the funeral in a short-sleeved shirt. It was freezing out. Many older people don't recognize feeling cold. She kept insisting she was fine.

We encouraged her to put on a coat, but she kept refusing. In a last attempt, I took out a heavy sweater that Bob often wore and told her if she put it on she would feel Bob putting his arms around her.

She accepted the idea and it became hers. She wore that sweater all through the winter. It comforted her. Sometimes, it helps to wear clothing or a piece of jewelry that the loved person used. It helps to have something physical to hold on to.

The need for acquiring a sweater or a ring sometimes leads to misunderstandings between family members. It may appear to be avaricious, though often friends and family really just want to hang on to the person they cared about.

When Bob died, one son wanted his cane. Another wanted his photography vest. A little bit of Bob left with each of them. I felt relieved to know that, though the closet was empty, his personal belongings were in loving hands.

Our behavior can run the gamut of irrationality during mourning. Some of us forget things. We start for the kitchen and can't remember that we started out to scramble eggs. It is not senility; it is mourning. Well-meaning friends often tell us that keeping busy helps. Sometimes it does and sometimes it doesn't.

Mourning is a time of insomnia. Trying to make decisions when you have been up all night leads to blunders. Be gentle with yourself. Let the pain be. Understand how difficult it is to stop searching for the person you loved. It seems that the harder you try to bring them back, the farther away they become.

In C.S. Lewis's book, *In a Grief Observed*, he wrote, "It is when I feel the least sorrow—getting into my morning bath is one of them—that my wife rushes upon my mind in her full reality, her otherness. This is good and tonic."

Forget a timetable. Only you will know when you are ready to let go of the pain and anxiety. Listen to your heart. It will let you know what to do.

My friend Mary Ellen Siegel nursed her husband through a long and difficult illness. Many acquaintances encouraged her to place him in a nursing home. "He has Alzheimer's. He won't know the difference," they said.

She answered, "He may not know, but I know." That was the only decision she could make, but someone else might find a nursing home the better choice.

Mary Ellen continued, "When I look in the mirror, I may see wrinkles and I may see thinning hair, but I never see guilt!"

Regret is a wasteful use of time. So is guilt. Yet too many of us suffer with both. We said or should have said something other than what we said. We did or didn't do what our instincts warned us to do.

We all make mistakes. We are all human and we are survivors. We punish ourselves with regret. We immobilize ourselves with guilt. Either way is a waste of living. Life is too short for that sort of indulgence.

There comes a time when the papers are signed, the closet has been emptied, and friends stop calling to see if you are OK. You are finally on your own. Welcome to your new world.

I have always had directional dyslexia. If someone puts up a new gas station, I don't recognize my way to the supermarket. Bob did most of the driving, and if I got behind the wheel he would coach me in a joking way. My confusions amused him. I'd never realized how often he filled in for my inadequacies. I seemed to be frozen in place. If I wanted to get somewhere, I had to do the driving.

Oh, how I missed the person who simply and easily filled in my gaps. When chairs needed to be set up, he'd do it. When light bulbs needed changing, he changed them. When I forgot to put the bread on the table, it appeared magically. He was a man who remembered. I was a woman who forgot.

In spite of all that, I'd always thought of myself as independent. Surely I was the one who maintained and sustained our relationship. Wrong!

I recognized all too clearly just how much he contributed. And I had to stop relying on his help. He was gone. It wasn't supposed to be that way. I felt angry with him for leaving me to cope on my own.

I knew I had to make an effort to prove to myself that I could make it on my own. With clenched teeth and wavering resolve, I decided to take a bike trip through the Netherlands. I'd always wanted to see the tulip fields in bloom.

I wasn't brave enough to travel totally on my own, so I decided to go under the auspices of Elderhostel. It would be a new beginning. Bob always said, "Courage is when you are afraid of something and you do it anyway." I was determined I would get back into the swim (or on to the wheel) of life.

I discovered something wonderful during the course of this adventure. As I let go, I found Bob was there with me in spirit. I knew it the night we listened to a lecture on the whys and wherefores of dike building. I had never been interested in engineering yet found myself fascinated. I sat there absorbed in every word. It was as if I were listening with Bob's ears and seeing with Bob's eyes.

One way of resolving grief incorporates habits and attitudes of your lost loved one into your new life.

Here I was looking at bridges, tunnels, and dikes and marveling at the construction. I never did that before.

I found myself watching men working on scaffolds. I stopped at building sites and stood transfixed by derricks. I saw what Bob saw, not as intelligently, not with his comprehension, but I saw with his heart. He will always be with me.

Integration

Sigmund Freud says in his book, *The Ego and the Id,* that you detach from the libido what you have invested in your loved one only when you reinstate it in your ego.

Karl Abraham in his *Short Study of the Development of the Libido, Selected Papers* declares, "The love object is not gone for now I carry it within myself and can never lose it."[33]

The most important task in mourning is internalizing the person you love and allowing him or her to become a part of your inner self. It takes time. In the beginning one remains connected to the external presence of the person who has died. As internalization takes place the loss becomes easier to bear.

You find you can discuss memories. You can manage thinking and sharing your feelings with others. At last you can come to grips with ambivalence. The inner and outer worlds synchronize.

In the process of mourning, the same defense a little child uses to quiet his fear of losing his mother surfaces. The child incorporates the idea of his mother into his ego so as not to lose her. He forms an inner picture of her in order to quell his separation anxiety. This enables him to form attachments. The adult mourner does exactly the same thing. Incorporation is a sign of a healthy personality. It is a sign of moving on. Welcome it. This is a time of growth and irrationality. It can be a time of immobilization or can be the moment to try something you have never done. If you let the exploration and consideration flow and accept that you are now a different person than you have ever been before, new projects will seem to present themselves from nowhere.

I thought of dying my hair red, buying a horse, moving to Alaska. Crazy, but the act of conceptualizing can be fun. Lightening up and grabbing for life is a path to healing.

A Word of Caution

Widows and widowers often try to fill the void by becoming involved in a new relationship too quickly.

Go slow. Having fun is great, but jumping into a commitment before coming to grips with your aloneness often leads to a poor choice in partners. Many therapists advise that you not make any important life change for at least a year.

One last exercise that may help you to sort things out is called a role diagram. A role can be anything that the self learns to do and can be tangible or intangible, emotional or concrete. We each have designated social roles such as mother, daughter, or police officer. Often we base our self-esteem on the way we function in those assignments. Relinquishing a job title may devastate or liberate us.

For years, I'd volunteered on an emergency hotline. I couldn't do that anymore. A friend's suggestion that I needed to keep busier infuriated me.

Each morning, I would make up my mind to get going, but time kept slipping by.

Creating my own role diagram and identifying my roles finally helped me see that I needed to break the routine and try something totally different. I decided on the bike trip. Even if it seems like a great effort, try the following exercise and see where it leads you.

Roles

On a large piece of paper draw circles to label your roles.[34] Below are some samples. Feel free to add your own.

1. Physical
   - → Sleeper _____
   - → Eater _____
   - → Sufferer _____
   - → My Role _____

2. Social-Familial
   - → Party–giver _____
   - → Mom/Dad _____
   - → Friend _____
   - → My Role _____

3. Professional
   - → Teacher _____
   - → Volunteer _____
   - → Artist _____
   - → My Role _____

4. Philosophical
   - → Religious _____
   - → Existentialist _____
   - → Pragmatist _____
   - → My Role _____

Put down your roles in the order you play them out and in terms of frequency and intensity.

Next to the roles, jot down your feelings about the role (angry, sad, happy). Put down whatever occurs to you. Don't censor anything.

Put a plus sign next to anything you feel good about. Put a check (✔) next to the role that is unsatisfying.

Sit with your chart for a few minutes. Then begin with one role and analyze it completely.

What is there about this role that needs reframing? Is there someone who can assist you in bringing that about? How do you feel about asking for help with it?

Address what stops you from accepting the role or the possibility of role change.

What will make you feel better about the situation?

Ask yourself what you need to do in order to let go of any impasse.

Let go. Allow yourself to feel whatever you feel.

Remember criticism is never helpful. Be gentle with yourself.

Your goal is to understand and set priorities. This is difficult work. Remind yourself to breathe as you do it. Life is precious.

Carpe diem. Seize the day, and live it fully.

My grandmother was a very wise woman. She used to tell me, "There will always be light and there will always be shadow. It is our task to live it all with gusto. It is our goal to handle it all with dignity."

Just remember that the one constant we have in life is that it is always changing. There is always another chapter in the making and always another lesson to be learned. Life is a journey. Vulnerability is the necessary baggage of showing up. I hope you will carry it well as you carry on.

Showing Up

As months go by
Memories stay
I place my feet
On the floor
Anyway

I go on
I go on

And then one day
I discover
A strength
Never known
All my own

I go on
I go on

I can stay
In my power
For an hour or more
By chanting
A mantra

I go on
I go on

That was then
This is after
It is new
It is real
And I feel

I go on
I go on

Maryann Schacht

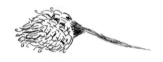

References

1. Jung, Carl. *Man & Symbols.* London: Aldres Books, 1984.

2. Harris, Thomas A., M.D. *I'm OK—You're OK.* New York: Harper and Row, 1967.

3. Pert, Candace. "Tomorrow's Medicine Today." *National Institutes of Mental Health, 57,* Bethesda, MD, (1989).

4. Cleeland, Charles S., M.D. "Pain Inventory." Pain Research Group, University of Wisconsin Medical School.

5. Cowles, Jane, Ph.D. *Pain Relief.* Master Media Publishing Corp., 1993.

6. Rossi, Ernest & Cheek, David. *Mind Body Therapy.* New York: W. W. Norton, 1988.

7. Bresler, David E., Ph.D, L.Ac. "Glove Anesthesia." 1995. See also *Free Yourself from Pain.* New York: Simon and Schuster, 1979.

8. Xiezu, Bian. *Essentials of Chinese Acupuncture.* Beijing: Foreign Language Press, 1980.

9. J.R. Worsley. *Is Acupuncture for You?* New York: Harper Collins, 1973.

10. Hippocrates, 400 B.C.

11. McDougall, John, M.D. *New McDougall Cookbook.* New York: Dutton, 1993.

12. Kempner, Walter, M.D. "The Rice Diet." Durham, North Carolina: Duke University Medical Center.

13. Pritikin, Nathan, M.D. *The Pritiken Promise.* New York: Bantam Books, 1991.

14. Ornish, Dean, M.D. *Eat More, Weigh Less.* New York: Harper Collins, 1993.

15. Wall, Steven, Ph.D. Biofeedback Training & Research Center in Cotati, CA.

16. Combrinck Graham, Lee, Ph.D. *Journal of Psychotherapy and Family 5* (1989).

17. Levinson, D.J., Ph.D. *The Seasons of Man's Life.* New York: Alfred Knopf, 1978.

18. Hale, Ann E. *Conducting Clinical Sociometric Explorations.* Roanoke: Royal Publishing Co., 1981.

19. Moreno, J.L., M.D. *Moreno's Social Atom, Sociometry, Experimental Method and the Science of Society.* Beacon, New York: Beacon House, 1951.

20. Van der May, James. "A Perceptual Social Atom Sociogram." *Group Psychotherapy and Psychodrama* 28 (1975).

21. Keleman, Stanley. *Living Your Dying.* New York: Random House, 1974.

22. Kaplan, Helen S., M.D., Ph.D. *The Illustrated Manual of Sex Therapy.* New York: Brunner/Mazel, 1987.

23. Berne, E. *Games People Play.* New York: Grove Press, 1964.

24. McGladrey & Pullen, LLP, Accountants, Bloomington, Minnesota, 1994.

25. Gibson, McIver Joan. "Values History Form." University of New Mexico, Albuquerque, NM.

26. Dossey, Larry, M.D. "What Is Prayer?" *Healing Beyond the Body.* Boston: Shambhala, 2003.

27. Benor, Daniel, M.D. "Survey of Spiritual Healing Research." *Complementary Medical Research* 4, no.1 (1990).

28. Koenig, Harold, M.D. *The Healing Power of Faith.* New York: Simon and Schuster, 1999.

29. Harris, William; Gowda, M. Kolb; Strychacz, C.P. "St. Luke's Hospital Study." Kansas City, MO.

30. Barry, J. "General and Comparative Study of the Psychokinetic Effect on Fungus Culture." *Journal of Parapsychology* 32 (1968).

31. Oxman, Thomas. "Positive Therapeutic Effects of Intercessory Prayer in a Coronary Care Unit Population." *Southern Medical Journal Vol.* 81, No. 7 (July 1988).

32. Israeli Study: "Scientific Proof Prayer Works." *Science and Spirit Magazine.* Texas Diocese of Holy Orthodox Church, 2002.

33. Abraham, Karl. *Selected Papers on Psycho-analysis.* London: Hogarth Press, 1924.

34. Starr, Adaline. *Rehearsal for Living.* Chicago: Nelson Hall, 1977.

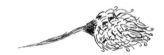

About the Author

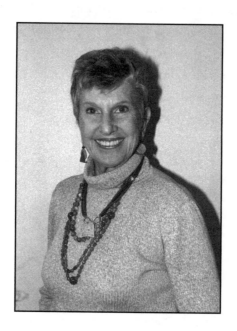

Maryann Schacht, MSW, BCD, is a psychotherapist whose diverse experience includes theater, radio commentary, psychodrama, family therapy, and imagery training, In private practice for over twenty-five years, she has facilitated groups at Kaiser Permanente, the American Cancer Society, and both Jewish and Catholic Family Services. She has presented at the American Society of Group Psychotherapy and Psychodrama, The American Educational Theater Association, and the National Association of Social Workers. She holds a Master's degree in Clinical Social Work from Columbia University and is Board Certified by the American Board of Examiners in Clinical Social Work.

Ms. Schacht lives in Santa Rosa, California, and has four sons, three stepsons, and ten grandchildren.

www.caregivers-challenge.net

I hope my book has helped you and answered your questions about the tough role of caregiving.

The first thing all caregivers learn is how constantly everything changes. We also know that each day brings new questions, new situations, and new trials. The person closest to the patient has a completely different view than the folks who drop in for a visit. Caregivers are often at the mercy of an inner critic who keeps hammering away at them. "Not doing enough." "Not up to the job." "You should…. Should…. Should…." Sharing what is happening in your life with others who are living your role offers you perspective. Reading the way other families are keeping their discussions open makes a difference in alleviating stress. You do not have to do it all. There are ways of lightening your load and finding respite.

I've designed my website, www.caregivers-challenge.net, to offer an avenue to the most current information on caregivers' resources. If contact information for important resources changes, the website will offer you the new information. If I discover a great new resource for caregivers, you'll find it on the website. I'll also announce events that I think will interest caregivers on the site.

When you yourself facing new and difficult questions, write to me. My site offers the link. Ask me and I will do my best to answer. If I don't have the answer, I'll help you find someone who does. I promise to treat all questions and answers with complete confidentiality.

Caregiving can feel like one of the loneliest jobs in the world. You have an opportunity to join an online community of people who are facing similar experiences and issues at http://www.caregivers-challenge.net. I hope you'll visit there soon. Let me know your reactions and suggestions. We will learn from each other.

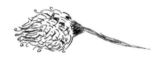

Order Form

Feterson Press
6477 Timber Springs Drive
Santa Rosa, CA 95409
phone: 707-537-9419
email: askmaryann@caregivers-challenge.net

Please send ____ copies of
A *Caregiver's Challenge: Living, Loving, Letting Go* at $16.95 each.

Please include $3.95 shipping and handling for the first copy
and $1.00 for each additional copy.
Californians please include 7.7% sales tax.

_____ Number of copies
_____ California Sales Tax
_____ Subtotal
_____ Shipping and Handling
_____ Total Enclosed

Name _____
Address _____
City _____ State _____ Zip _____
Email _____

Visit our website at www.caregivers-challenge.net

Printed in the United States
Code Numbers

ISBN 0-9764140-0-7

51695>

9 780976 414001